AF730631

Physeo

TABLE OF CONTENTS

NEUROLOGY......6

Section 1: Ischemic Stroke......6
Section 2: Cerebral Venous Thrombosis......12
Section 3: Movement Disorders: Parkinson & Huntington Disease......15
Section 4: Movement Disorders: Tremor & Ataxia......18
Section 5: Movement Disorders: Restless Leg Syndrome & Tourette Syndrome......21
Section 6: Meningitis......23
Section 7: Encephalitis......26
Section 8: Brain Abscess & Spinal Epidural Abscess......27
Section 9: Dementia......30
Section 10: Altered Mental Status......37
Section 11: Demyelinating Disease......41
Section 12: Neuromuscular Disease......45
Section 13: Neurofibromatosis Type I, II and Tuberous Sclerosis......50
Section 14: Neurocutaneous Syndromes: Sturge-Weber and von-Hippel-Lindau Syndromes......54
Section 15: Anterior Cord Syndrome, Central Cord Syndrome & Brown-Sequard Syndrome......57
Section 16: Cauda Equina Syndrome, Syringomyelia & Transverse Myelitis......60
Section 17: Poliomyelitis, Amyotrophic Lateral Sclerosis & Horner Syndrome......63
Section 18: Seizures: Causes, Types, and Workup......66
Section 19: Seizures: Differential Diagnosis and Management......69
Section 20: Aphasia and Neglect......72
Section 21: Localizing Neurologic Lesions: Introduction......75
Section 22: Cerebral Cortex, Subcortex, Brainstem and Cerebellum......76
Section 23: Spinal Cord, Peripheral Neurons, Neuromuscular Junction, Muscles, Diagnosis & Management......80
Section 24: Intracranial Hemorrhage: Subdural & Epidural Hematoma......83
Section 25: Intracranial Hemorrhage: Subarachnoid & Intraparenchymal Hemorrhage......87
Section 26: Headaches......91
Section 27: Nervous System Tumors: Gliomas, Pilocytic Astrocytoma, GB Multiforme......95
Section 28: Nervous System Tumors: Oligodendroglioma & Ependymoma......99
Section 29: Schwannoma, Medulloblastoma, Hemangioblastoma......101
Section 30: Meningioma, Sellar & Suprasellar Tumor & Secondary Brain Tumors......104
Section 31: Dizziness & Vertigo......108
Section 32: Syncope......113

TABLES & FIGURES......115

We would like to extend a special thanks to the following individuals who have spent countless hours and support to make Physeo possible.

Ajay Davidson, MD

Alexandra Galel, MD

Alexandra Harding

Anissa Laine Bayabos Amilhamja

Anne-Sophie van Wingerden
Medical Student
Columbia Vagelos College of Physicians and Surgeons

Antonio Acevedo

Ayan Agarwal
MBBS Student
Vardhman Mahavir Medical College and Safdarjung Hospital
New Delhi, India

Brianna Cocuzzo, MsC

Brooke Walsh, MS

Camelita Thrift

Christopher A. Price, MS

Genevieve Saliuk
MD Candidate 2024
UTMB School of Medicine

George Myo Win, BS
University of Missouri-Columbia School of Medicine

Ghadeer Magdy Elshafey, MD

H. Robert Cannon, DO

Dr. Jabran Wasti, House Officer
Dr. Ruth K.M. Pfau Civil Hospital
Karachi, Pakistan

Jae Cheol Bae

Dr. James Nunn

Jennifer M. Locke, BA
MD Candidate

Justin Wong, DO

Kurestin Miller, BA
MD Candidate

Lauren S. Faber, MD

Lauren Schwartz

Lee Azolai

Leslie Jewett, MD

Logan B. Carlyle, OMS-II

Marisol Cárdenas Calderón, MD

Mark Parry, MD, Resident Physician
Department of Obstetrics and Gynecology
OhioHealth – Riverside Methodist
Columbus, Ohio

Mason T. Bennet

Mateo Betancourt Escobar
Universidad Autónoma de San Luis
Potosí, Mexico

Mohamed Elshennawy

Natalia Kerr, MD

Nijat Aliyev, MD

Nikoloz Karazanashvili

Nirupamaa Sivanushanthan
Medical Student

Ostapenko Karolina

Dr. Rahil Patel, Medical Officer
Sharda Hospital
New Delhi, India

Mr. Rishabh Goyal

Roaa Zayat, MD

Rojin Arefi, MD

Ryan Zia

Salikh Murtaliev, MD

Sarah Jaber, D.O.
Internal Medicine Physician

Sergio R. Ortiz, MD, MPH

Shawna-Kay Young
MD Student

Shelia Chandrahas

Soomal Zukhruf Memon

Sumit Raut

Syed Ali Haider

Syed Awais Ahmed, MD

Tori Walsh

Tamari Papidze

Telyn Peterson, OMS-III
Rocky Vista University
Southern Utah

Trey Edwards, DO

Warda Hameed, MD

Yasmeen Abdulrahman, MD

Yomna Dean, MS-4

Zurabi Zaalishvili, MD

NEUROLOGY

Neurology | Section 1: Ischemic Stroke

I. Ischemic Stroke: Definition
  A. Acute neurological condition caused by disruption of blood flow to the brain
  B. More common than hemorrhagic stroke
  C. Symptoms last > 24 hours (vs. transient ischemic attack)

II. Ischemic Stroke: Risk Factors
  A. Non-modifiable risk factors
    1. Age ≥ 65 years
    2. Male gender
    3. Family history of stroke and cardiovascular disease
    4. History of transient ischemic attack (TIA)
  B. Modifiable risk factors
    1. Hypertension (strongest risk factor)
    2. Hyperlipidemia
    3. Carotid artery atherosclerosis
    4. Atrial fibrillation
    5. Tobacco use

III. Ischemic Stroke: Etiology
  A. Thrombotic stroke: most common
    1. Rupture of atherosclerotic plaque in cerebral vessel → exposure of subendothelial collagen → thrombus occluding vascular lumen
    2. Risk factors: hypertension, atherosclerosis
    3. Fluctuating symptoms with periods of improvement
    4. Large vessel: occlusion at branching point
    5. Small vessel: lacunar infarct affecting deep brain structures
  B. Embolic stroke
    1. Cardiac emboli: atrial fibrillation, rheumatic heart disease, infective endocarditis, ventricular aneurysm
    2. Atheroemboli: internal carotid artery
    3. Paradoxical emboli: atrial septal defect, patent foramen ovale
    4. Most commonly affects middle cerebral artery (MCA)
    5. Abrupt onset of symptoms with maximal intensity at onset
  C. Global cerebral ischemia
    1. Diffuse cerebral hypoperfusion: shock or bilateral carotid artery atherosclerosis
    2. Commonly causes watershed infarct: infarction of the most distal areas of vascular territories
      a) ACA/MCA watershed infarct; MCA/PCA watershed infarct
      b) Between deep and superficial MCA branches

IV. Ischemic Stroke: Clinical Presentation
  A. Weakness
  B. Paralysis
  C. Aphasia
  D. Impaired consciousness
  E. Headache
  F. Seizures
  G. Nausea and vomiting
  H. MCA stroke
    1. Weakness and sensory loss in contralateral lower face and upper extremity
    2. Dysphagia, dysarthria, and aphasia
  I. ACA stroke
    1. Weakness and sensory loss in contralateral lower extremity
  J. ACA/MCA watershed stroke
    1. Proximal upper and lower extremity weakness sparing distal extremities ("man-in-the-barrel syndrome")
  K. MCA/PCA watershed stroke
    1. Visual disturbances and visual hallucinations
  L. Lacunar stroke
    1. Pure motor stroke: infarct in posterior limb of internal capsule; unilateral motor deficits with no sensory, visual or higher cortical dysfunction
    2. Pure sensory stroke: infarct in VPL thalamic nucleus; unilateral sensory loss affecting face, arm and leg
    3. Ataxic hemiparesis: infarct in anterior limb of internal capsule; ipsilateral hand and leg incoordination with weakness
    4. Dysarthria-clumsy hand syndrome: infarct in basis pontis; hand weakness and motor aphasia
  M. Thalamic stroke
    1. Contralateral hemiparesis and sensory loss
    2. Miotic unreactive pupil with gaze deviation away from the affected side
  N. Medial medullary stroke (Dejerine syndrome)
    1. Contralateral spastic weakness
    2. Contralateral loss of vibration and proprioception
    3. Tongue deviation ipsilateral to the lesion
  O. Lateral medullary stroke (Wallenberg syndrome)
    1. Hoarseness, dysphagia, ipsilateral Horner syndrome
    2. Contralateral loss of pain and temperature sensation

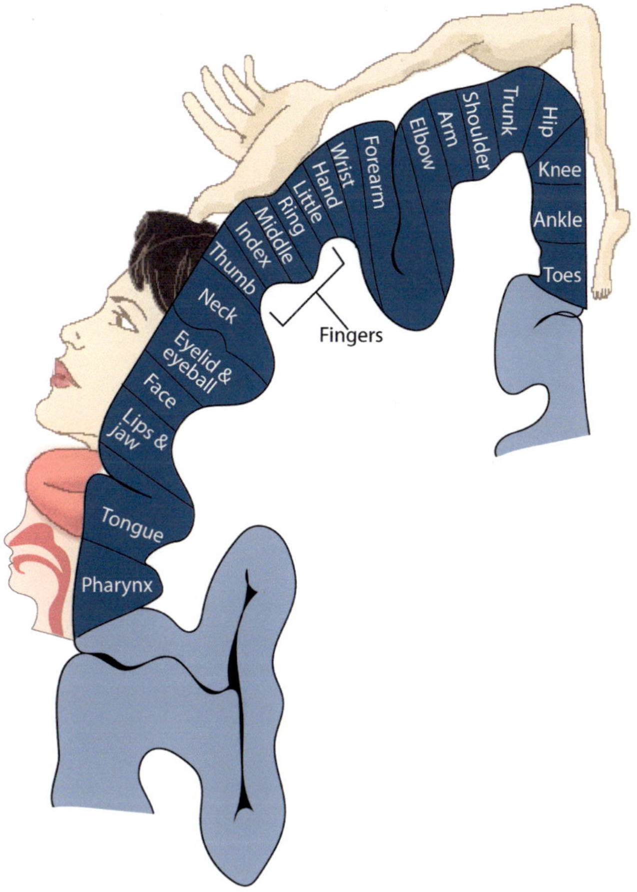

FIGURE 13.1.1 - The Cerebral Homunculus

Stroke	Key Features
MCA stroke	- Dysphagia, dysarthria, aphasia - Weakness and sensory loss in contralateral lower face and arm
ACA stroke	- Weakness and sensory loss in contralateral lower extremity
ACA/MCA watershed stroke	- Proximal upper and lower extremity weakness ("Man-in-the-barrel syndrome")
MCA/PCA watershed stroke	- Visual disturbances and visual hallucinations
Lacunar stroke	- Pure motor stroke (posterior limb of internal capsule) - Pure sensory stroke (ventroposterolateral nucleus of thalamus) - Ataxic hemiparesis (anterior limb of internal capsule) - Dysarthria-clumsy hand syndrome (basis pontis)
Thalamic stroke	- Contralateral hemiparesis and sensory loss
Medial medullary stroke	- Contralateral spastic weakness - Contralateral loss of vibration and proprioception - Tongue deviation ipsilateral to the lesion
Lateral medullary stroke	- Hoarseness, dysphagia - Ipsilateral Horner syndrome - Contralateral loss of pain and temperature sensation

TABLE 13.1.1 - Types of Stroke

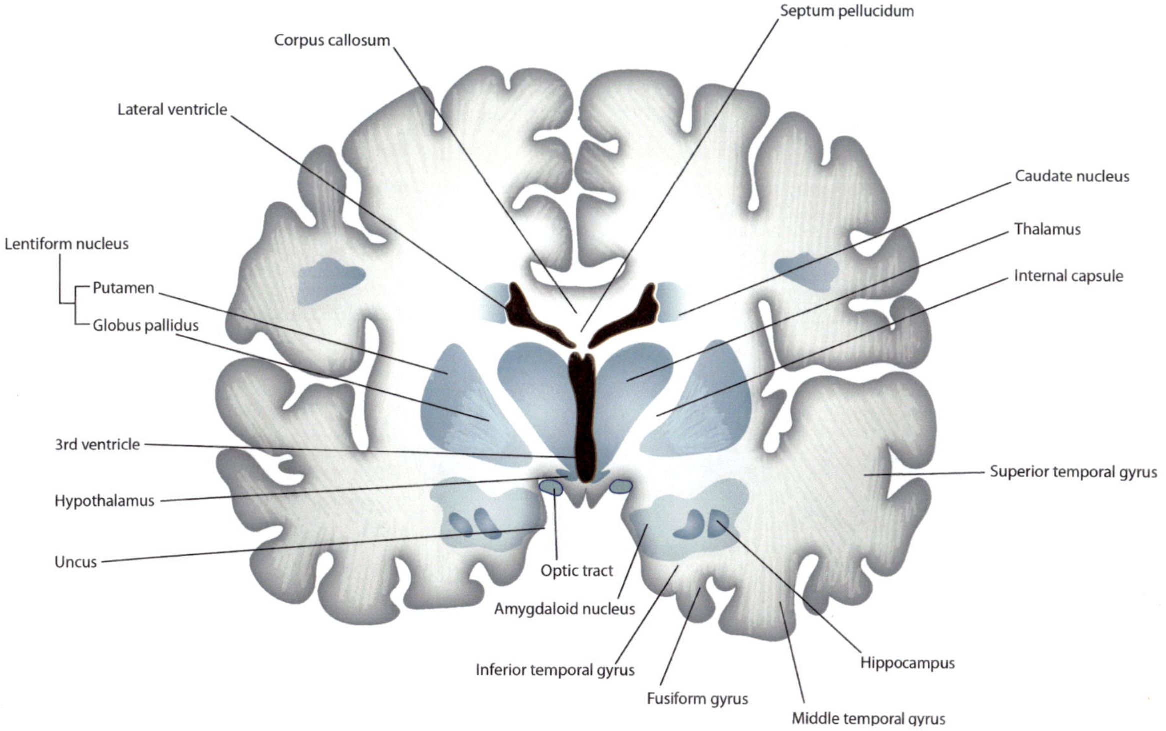

FIGURE 13.1.2 - The Deep Brain Structures

V. Ischemic Stroke: Diagnosis
   A. Determine the time elapsed from onset of symptoms
   B. Non-contrast head CT scan (first-line imaging)
      1. To rule out intracranial hemorrhage prior to thrombolytic administration
      2. Detects ischemic changes ~ 6 hours after symptom onset
      3. Hypodense area of necrosis
      4. Loss of corticomedullary differentiation and effacement of sulci
   C. Diffusion-weighted MRI
      1. Ischemic changes can be detected ~ 3 minutes after symptom onset
      2. More time-consuming and more expensive than CT scan
      3. Indicated in case of high suspicion of stroke with normal head CT results
   D. CT angiography
      1. Identifies the occluded vessel
   E. Indications
      1. High index of suspicion for stroke with negative CT and MRI results
      2. Patient cannot receive thrombolytic therapy but is eligible for mechanical thrombectomy
   F. Other studies
      1. Serum glucose
      2. Complete blood count
      3. ECG and serum troponin
      4. Urine drug screen
      5. Carotid ultrasound and TTE/TEE
      6. Coagulation panel (PT/INR, PTT) ordered immediately

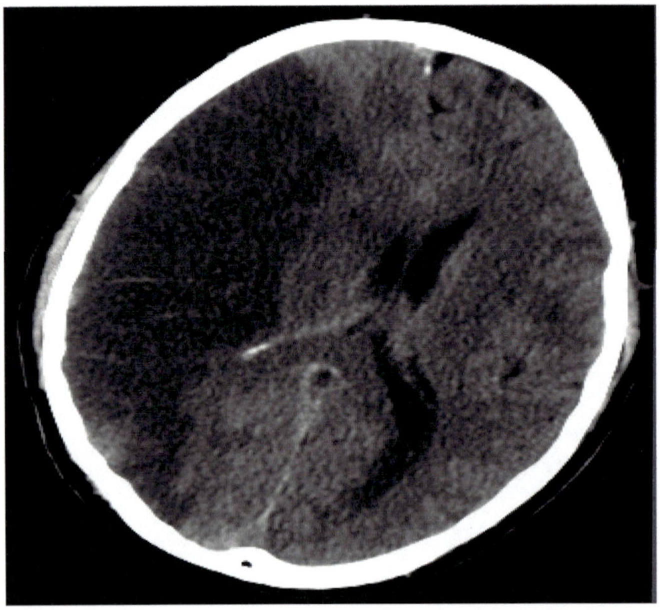

FIGURE 13.1.3 - CT Scan of the Head: Ischemic Stroke

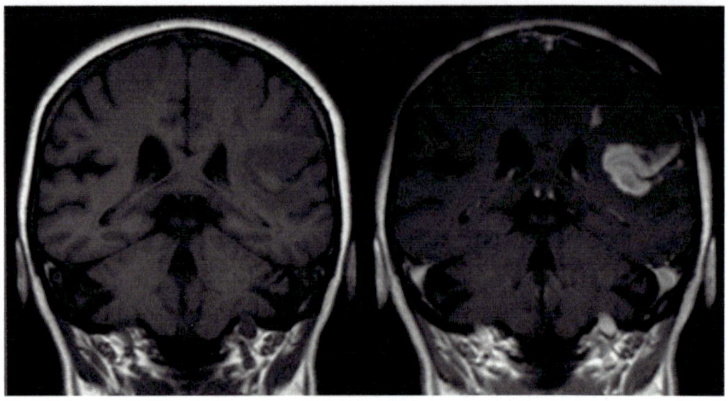

FIGURE 13.1.4 - MRI of the Brain: Ischemic Stroke

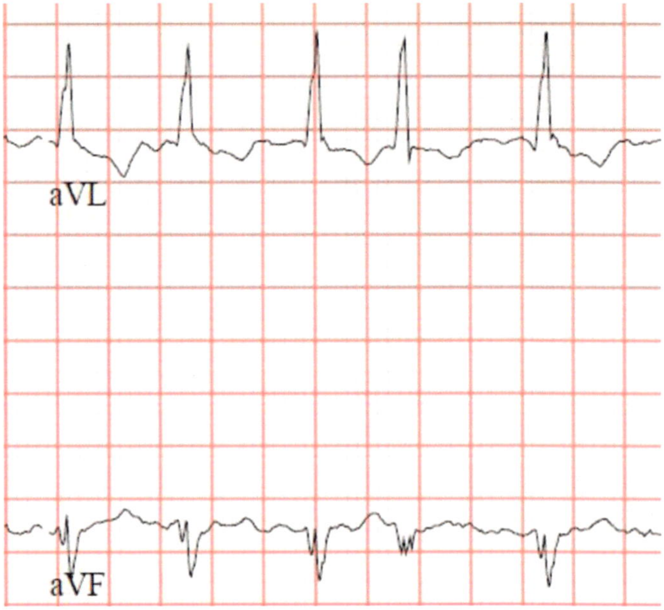

FIGURE 13.1.5 - ECG: Atrial Fibrillation

VI. Ischemic Stroke: Management
   A. Dual antiplatelet therapy: aspirin and clopidogrel
   B. IV thrombolytic therapy (tPA)
      1. Administered in acute ischemic stroke after excluding intracranial hemorrhage
      2. Time elapsed from symptoms onset: 3-4.5 hours
      3. Complications: intracranial or extracranial bleeding
   C. Strict exclusion criteria for thrombolytic therapy
      1. History of intracranial hemorrhage, tumor, vascular malformation
      2. Head trauma or stroke in the past 3 months, recent intracranial surgery
      3. Hemorrhagic stroke, active internal bleeding
      4. Hypertension (> 185/110 mmHg), ↓ platelets (< 100,000 cells/mm^3)
      5. Blood glucose < 50 mg/dL, INR > 1.7, PT > 15 sec, PTT > 40 sec
   D. Mechanical thrombectomy
      1. Mechanical removal of thrombus through catheter inserted mostly via femoral artery
      2. For hemodynamically unstable patients or those with contraindications to thrombolytic therapy

E. Hypertensive patients
   1. ↑ Blood pressure usually tolerated in ischemic stroke patients; maintains mean arterial pressure necessary for cerebral perfusion
   2. If initial blood pressure is > 220/120 mmHg reduce it to < 185/110 mmHg before thrombolytic therapy

F. <u>CHA_2DS_2-VASc</u> score for risk stratification
   1. Total score of 0: low risk for stroke; no prophylaxis
   2. Total score of 1: intermediate risk for stroke; aspirin or anticoagulants
   3. Total score of ≥ 2: high risk for stroke; anticoagulants

Letter	Risk Factor	Score
C	Congestive Heart Failure (or LV systolic dysfunction)	1
H	Hypertension	1
A_2	Age ≥ 75 years	2
D	Diabetes mellitus	1
S_2	Stroke/TIA/Thromboembolism	2
V	Vascular disease (e.g. Peripheral arterial disease, Myocardial infarction, aortic plaque)	1
A	Age 65-74 years	1
Sc	Sex category (i.e. female sex)	1
	Maximum score	9

TABLE 13.1.2 - CHA_2DS_2-VASc Score

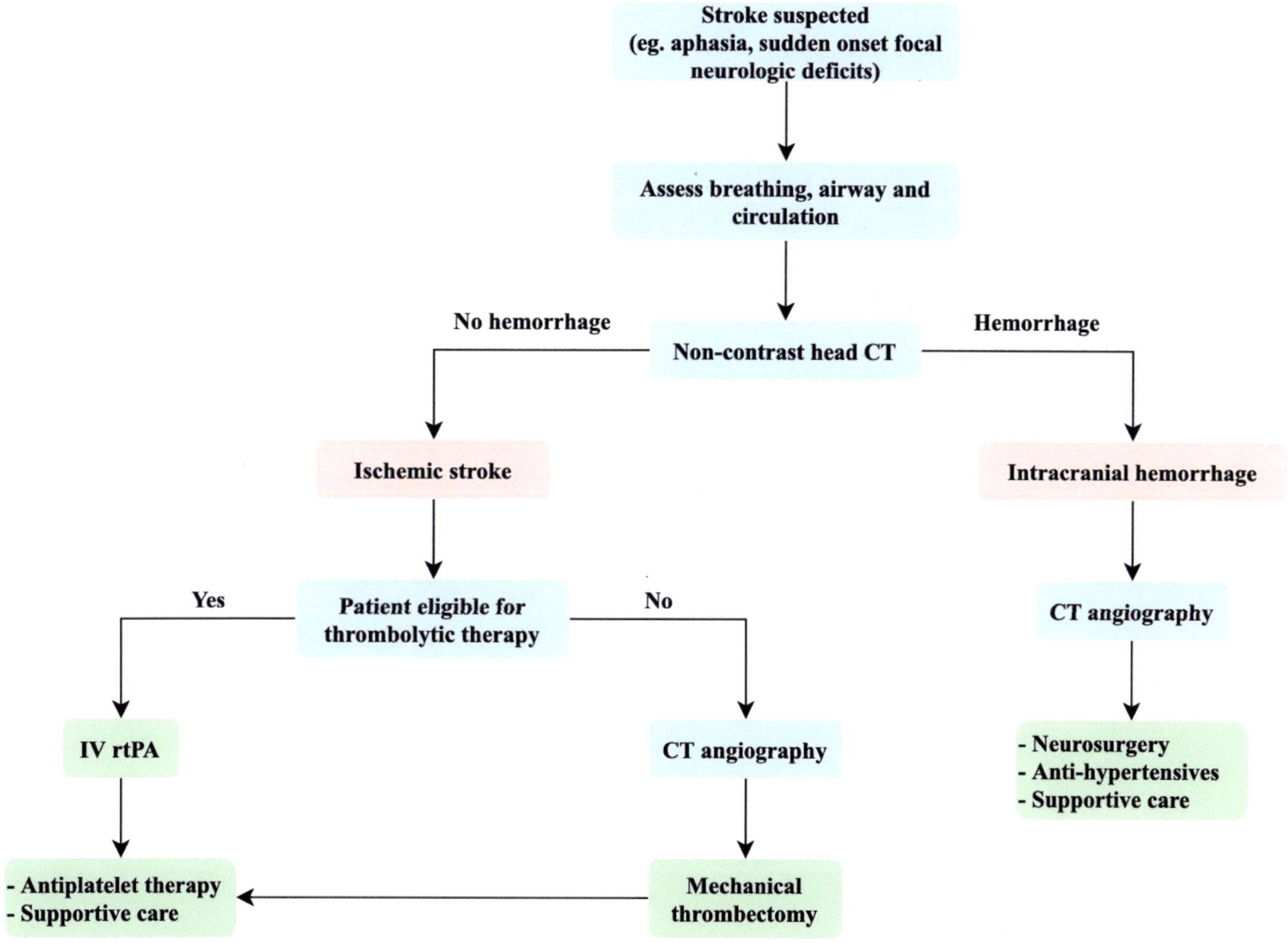

FIGURE 13.1.6 - Management of Stroke

REVIEW QUESTIONS

1. An 81-year-old man is brought o the emergency department because of slurred speech which started 20-minutes ago. He was watching TV when he suddenly felt weakness in his right hand. He called his wife, who then noticed his speech was slurred prompting her to call an ambulance. Past medical history is significant for uncontrolled hypertension for the last 20-years. He has been smoking 2-packs of cigarettes per day for 60-years. Physical exam shows weakness and sensory loss of his right lower face and right upper extremity. Laboratory studies show total cholesterol level of 300 mg/dL (150-240 mg/dL). What is the strongest risk factor for this patient's current condition?
   - **The strongest risk factor for this patient's current condition is hypertension.**
   - This patient presents with acute onset of slurred speech.
   - The physical exam shows weakness and sensory loss on his right lower face and right upper extremity.
   - This is a classic description of the left middle cerebral artery stroke.
   - The patient has multiple risk factors for ischemic stroke.
   - First, he has uncontrolled hypertension for the last 20 years. Additionally, he has been smoking 2 packs of cigarettes per day for 60 years. He also has hypercholesterolemia.
   - However, the strongest risk factor for any type of stroke is hypertension.

2. A 52-year-old woman is brought to the emergency department because of a headache and fatigue for 12-hours. She received low molecular weight heparin for an acute deep venous thrombosis 1-day ago. Physical examination shows weakness and sensory loss in the right lower extremity with hyperactive reflexes. Non-contrast head CT scan reveals hypodense parenchyma with loss of corticomedullary differentiation in the left anterior cerebral artery territory. There is no sign of intracranial hemorrhage. Which two cardiac conditions can account for this patient's current symptoms?
   - **ASD and PFO can account for this patient's current symptoms.**
   - This patient presents with a headache and fatigue.
   - Physical examination shows weakness and sensory loss in the right lower extremity with hyperactive reflexes.
   - She received low molecular weight heparin for acute deep venous thrombosis 1-day ago.
   - A non-contrast head CT scan shows hypodense parenchyma in the left anterior cerebral artery territory.
   - All of these clues suggest an ischemic stroke of the left anterior cerebral artery.
   - This patient had a thrombus in her peripheral veins that eventually ended up in the cerebral arteries.
   - Normally, a venous thrombus cannot bypass the lungs because it will become stuck in the pulmonary arteries or capillaries.
   - However, if there is an intracardiac right to left shunt, a venous thrombus can travel from the right atrium to the left atrium through this shunt and embolize to the brain. This phenomenon is known as paradoxical embolus.
   - Atrial septal defect and patent foramen ovale are two cardiac conditions that can account for paradoxical embolus.

REVIEW QUESTIONS

3. A 65-year-old man is brought to the emergency department because of acute loss of sensation to the right side of his body 30-minutes ago. Past medical history is significant for hypertension which is poorly controlled with lisinopril. Physical examination shows loss of pinprick sensation on the right-side of his body and left side of his face. He also has difficulty swallowing, hoarse voice, drooping of the left eyelid and miosis of the left pupil. What is the best next step in management for this patient?

- **The next best step is a non-contrast CT scan of the head.**
- This patient has acute loss of pinprick sensation on the right-side of his body and left-side of his face. He also has difficulty swallowing, and hoarse voice.
- Dysphagia in this case is most likely caused by damage to the glossopharyngeal and vagal nerve nuclei, while his hoarse voice is explained by damage solely to the vagal nucleus.
- The patient also has drooping of the left eyelid and miosis of the left pupil indicating left-sided Horner syndrome. Horner syndrome in this case is likely caused by damage to descending hypothalamic fibers.
- Considering all these clues, this patient most likely has a left lateral medullary stroke, also known as Wallenberg syndrome.

4. A 66-year-old man is brought to the emergency department because of slurred speech that started 2-hours ago. He was shoveling snow when he suddenly fell on the ground. Past medical history is significant for concussion due to motor vehicle accident 2- months ago. Vital signs include temperature of 36° C (96.8° F), blood pressure of 180/100 mmHg, and heart rate of 91 beats/min. Laboratory studies show platelet count of 120,000 cells/mm^3 (150,000-400,000 cells/mm^3). Non-contrast head CT scan reveals hypodense area with loss of corticomedullary differentiation in the right middle cerebral artery territory. A resident suggests thrombolytic therapy but the physician declines his suggestion. Which of the following makes this patient ineligible for pharmacological management of his current condition?

   A. Time since the onset of symptoms
   B. Past medical history
   C. Blood pressure
   D. Platelet count

- **The correct answer is option B.**
- This patient presents with acute-onset slurred speech that started 2-hours ago.
- Non-contrast head CT scan reveals hypodense area with loss of corticomedullary differentiation in the right middle cerebral artery territory.
- These findings are consistent with an ischemic stroke of the right middle cerebral artery.
- A resident suggests thrombolytic therapy but the physician declines his suggestion. The most likely reason behind this decision is that the patient has a past medical history of concussion due to a motor vehicle accident within the past 3-months.
- Head trauma within the past 3 months is a strict exclusion criterion for thrombolytic therapy.
- Option A is incorrect because thrombolytic therapy can be administered within the 4.5 hours after symptom onset. This patient's symptoms started 2 hours ago.
- Option C is incorrect because the blood pressure more than 185/110 mmHg is a strict exclusion criterion for thrombolytics. This patient has a blood pressure of 180/100 mmHg.
- Option D is incorrect because the platelet count less than 100,000 cells/mm^3 is the strict exclusion criterion for tPA. This patient, on the other hand, has a platelet count of 120,000 cells/mm^3.

Neurology | Section 2: Cerebral Venous Thrombosis

I. Cerebral Venous Thrombosis: Definition
   A. Thrombosis of cerebral veins or dural venous sinuses
   B. Anatomical location: can occur in any dural venous sinus
      1. Most common include transverse sinus and superior sagittal sinus
   C. Etiology
      1. Septic and non-septic cerebral venous thrombosis
   D. Females > males (3:1)

II. Cerebral Venous Thrombosis: Types
   A. Non-septic
      1. Hypercoagulability: malignancy, factor V Leiden, pregnancy, oral contraceptives, polycythemia, nephrotic syndrome
      2. Neurological procedures (e.g. lumbar puncture)
      3. Hyperhomocysteinemia
      4. Thrombotic thrombocytopenic purpura, sickle cell disease
   B. Septic
      1. Sinusitis or periorbital/orbital cellulitis
      2. Dental infections
      3. Mid-facial infections ("danger triangle")
      4. Acute otitis media
      5. Meningitis
   C. Cavernous sinus thrombosis
      1. Thrombotic occlusion of cavernous sinuses due to infection from "danger triangle"
   D. Specific findings
      1. Ophthalmoplegia (CN III, IV, VI)
      2. Horner syndrome (sympathetic fibers)
      3. ↓ corneal and maxillary sensation (CN V_1 and V_2)

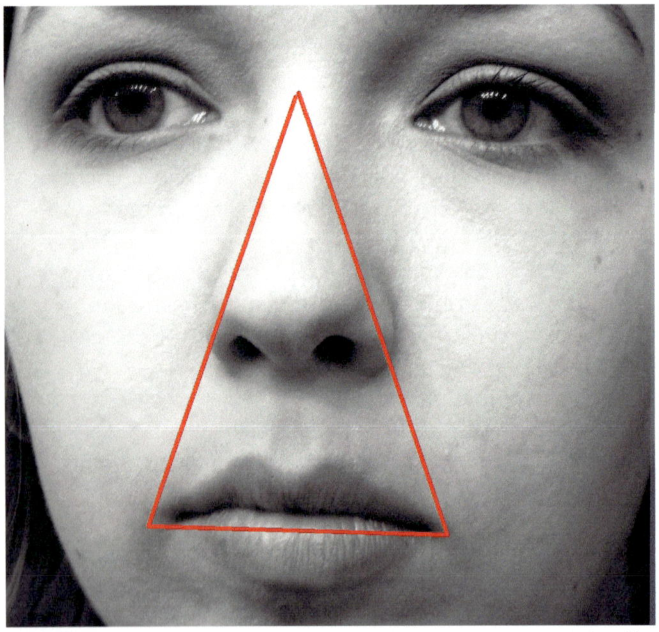

FIGURE 13.1.7 - The Danger Triangle

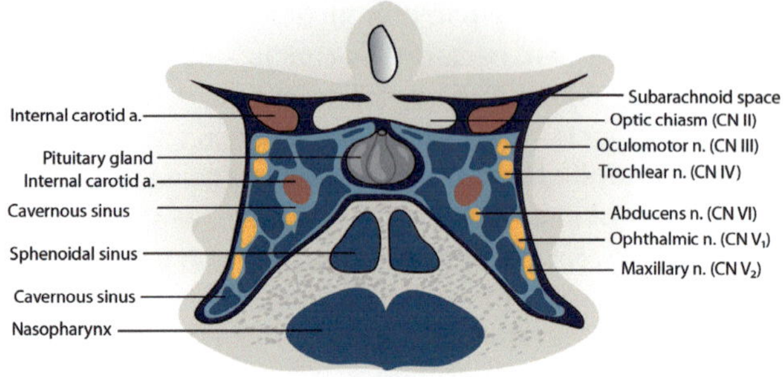

FIGURE 13.1.8 - The Cavernous Sinus

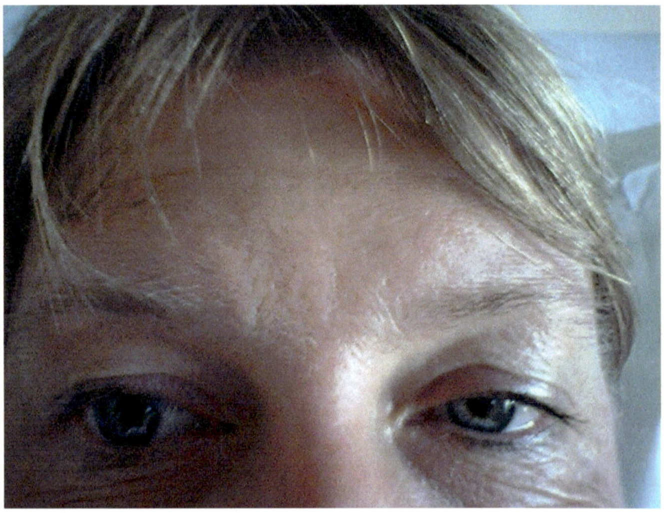

FIGURE 13.1.9 - Horner Syndrome

III. Cerebral Venous Thrombosis: Clinical Presentation
   A. Headache (most common)
   B. Possible seizures
   C. Intracranial hypertension
      1. Papilledema and diplopia
      2. Nausea and vomiting
   D. Cranial neuropathy
      1. Tinnitus, facial palsy, sensorineural hearing loss

IV. Cerebral Venous Thrombosis: Diagnosis
   A. Magnetic resonance venography (MRV): test of choice
   B. CT venography: if MRV is contraindicated or unavailable
   C. Findings in both
      1. Intraluminal venous thrombus
      2. Absence of blood flow
      3. "Empty delta" sign
   D. Lab
      1. D-dimer: usually elevated; low levels do not exclude cerebral venous thrombosis
      2. Coagulation panel (PT/INR, PTT)
      3. CBC, ESR and CRP
      4. Blood culture

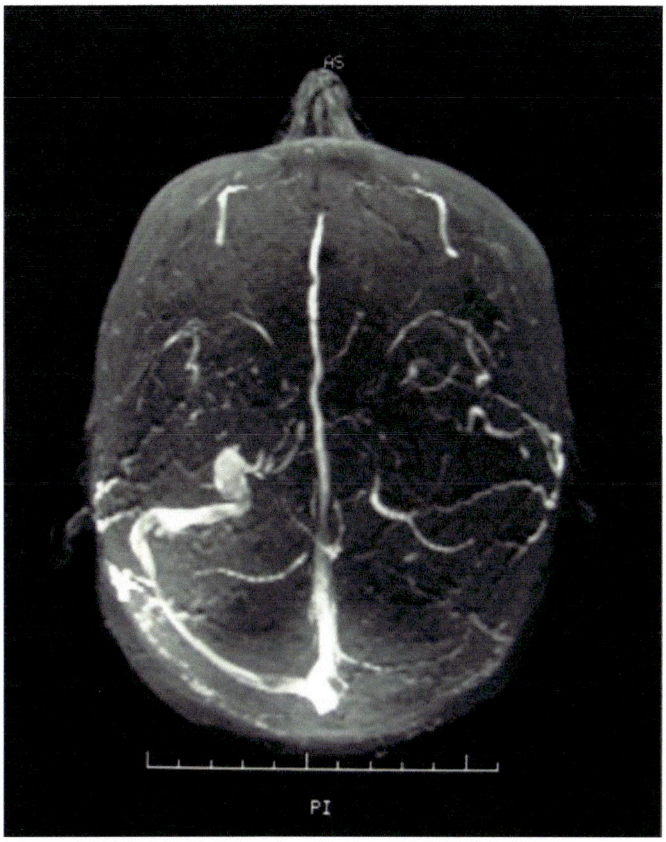

FIGURE 13.1.10 - MR Venography: Cerebral Venous Thrombosis

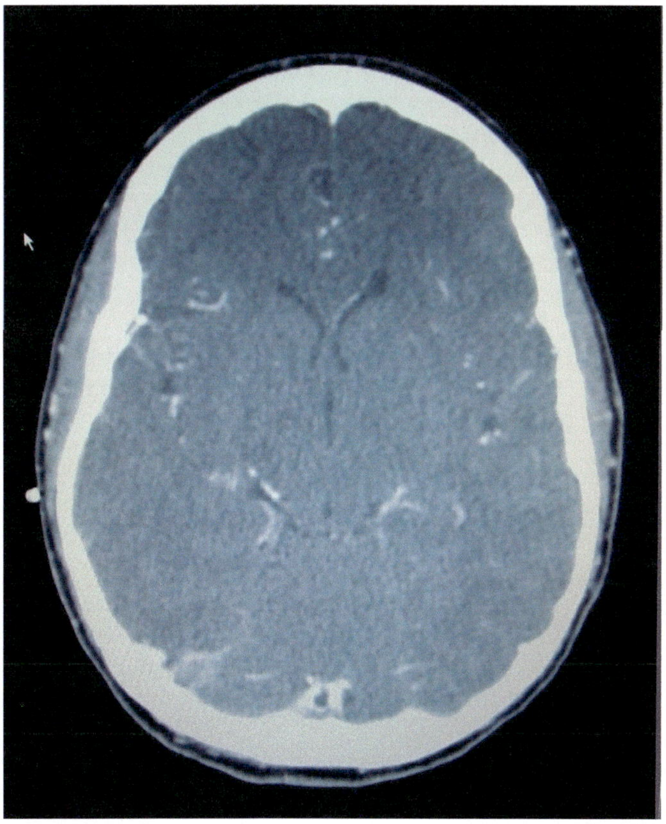

FIGURE 13.1.11 - CT Scan of Head: "Empty Delta" Sign

V. Cerebral Venous Thrombosis: Management
   A. Acute anticoagulation
      1. Low molecular weight heparin (LMWH): first-line
      2. Unfractionated heparin
      3. Chronic anticoagulation therapy: warfarin
   B. Antibiotic therapy (septic cerebral venous thrombosis)
      1. Vancomycin and ceftriaxone: staphylococcus
      2. Metronidazole: anaerobes

REVIEW QUESTIONS

1. A 25-year-old woman comes to the emergency room because of a severe headache and ringing in her ears for the last 2-days. She takes no medications and has no significant past medical history, however she mentions one week ago she was treated for a left maxillary periodontal abscess. Ophthalmic examination shows bilateral papilledema. Urine pregnancy test and serum beta-hCG are negative. Magnetic resonance venography shows diminished blood flow in the superior sagittal sinus. What risk factor most likely predisposed her to this condition?
   - **The most likely risk factor is a recent dental infection.**
   - This patient presents with a headache, and tinnitus.
   - Ophthalmic examination shows bilateral papilledema.
   - Magnetic resonance venography shows diminished blood flow in the superior sagittal sinus.
   - All of these findings are consistent with cerebral venous thrombosis.
   - Oral contraceptive use is also a risk factor for CVT however this patient does not take any medications. Therefore the most likely predisposing risk factor is the recent periodontal infection.

2. An 8-year-old boy is brought to the emergency department by his parents because of a severe headache for 4-days. His mother states the his headache has worsened over the past few days and the boy had an episode of emesis this morning. The boy is crying and states that he cant stop the ringing in his ears. Vital signs include temperature of 39° C (102.2° F), blood pressure of 100/80 mmHg, heart rate of 92 beats/min, and respiratory rate of 16 breaths/min. Ophthalmic examination shows bilateral papilledema. A non-contrast CT head is ordered and shows a hypodense mass with hyperdense borders and diminished blood flow in the inferior sagittal sinus. Which of the following is the best treatment option for this patient?

   A. Enoxaparin, vancomycin, and ceftriaxone
   B. Enoxaparin and aztreonam
   C. Unfractionated heparin
   D. Warfarin

   - **The correct answer is option A.**
   - This young boy presents with severe headache, vomiting, and tinnitus.
   - He recently finished a course of antibiotics for bacterial sinusitis.
   - Vital signs are remarkable for a fever of 39° C (102.2° F).
   - Ophthalmic examination shows bilateral papilledema indicating increased intracranial pressure.
   - Non-contrast head CT scan shows a hypodense mass with hyperdense borders and diminished blood flow in the inferior sagittal sinus.
   - These findings are suggestive of a cerebral venous thrombosis.
   - This patient likely has a septic cerebral venous thrombosis due to contiguous spread of infection from the paranasal sinuses.
   - All patients with cerebral venous thrombosis should receive acute anticoagulation, preferably with low molecular weight heparin such as enoxaparin.
   - Since this is a septic thrombosis, the patient should also receive the antibiotic coverage for *Staphylococcus* and gram negative bacteria.
   - Vancomycin and ceftriaxone will be helpful in this case.
   - Therefore, the patient should receive enoxaparin, vancomycin, and ceftriaxone.
   - Option B is incorrect because aztreonam does not cover Gram-positive bacteria. It only covers Gram-negative bacteria.
   - Option C is incorrect because low molecular weight heparin is preferred over unfractionated heparin for the initial management of cerebral venous thrombosis. Additionally, since this is the case of a septic cerebral venous thrombosis, the patient needs antibiotics.
   - Option D is incorrect because warfarin is used for chronic, rather than acute, anticoagulation in patients with cerebral venous thrombosis.

Neurology | Section 3: Movement Disorders: Parkinson & Huntington Disease

I. Parkinson Disease: Definition
- A. Neurodegenerative disorder
- B. Loss of dopaminergic neurons in substantia nigra
- C. Affects the elderly > 40 years of age

II. Parkinson Disease: Clinical Features
- **A.** **"TRAP"** symptoms
  - 1. Resting **T**remor "pill-rolling"
    - a) Typically affects one hand first (asymmetric)
    - b) The most common presenting symptom
  - **2.** **R**igidity: increased resistance to passive movement around a joint (lead-pipe or cogwheel rigidity)
  - **3.** **A**kinesia/bradykinesia
    - a) Generalized slowness and reduced ability to initiate movements (e.g. standing up from a chair)
    - b) Narrow-based, shuffling gait
    - c) Micrographia, hypomimia, hypophonia
  - **4.** **P**ostural instability (late manifestation)
    - a) Loss of centrally-mediated postural reflexes
    - b) Flexed axial posture, recurrent falls
- B. Mood disturbances (most commonly depression)
- C. Dementia (late manifestation): psychomotor retardation, memory impairment, altered personality
- D. Autonomic dysfunction: constipation, dysphagia, urinary and sexual disturbances

III. Parkinson Disease: Diagnosis
- A. Diagnosis is dependent on clinical findings
- B. There is no single test that can definitively diagnose Parkinson disease

IV. Parkinson Disease: Management
- A. Levodopa/carbidopa
  - 1. Moderate to severe symptoms, patients > 65 years of age
  - 2. Early side effects: nausea, dizziness, hallucinations, orthostatic hypotension
  - 3. Late side effects: dyskinesia (involuntary movements)
  - 4. "On-off" phenomenon: episodes of improved mobility "on-period" and impaired mobility "off-period"
- B. Dopamine agonists (e.g. pramipexole, ropinirole, bromocriptine)
  - 1. May be used for moderate to severe symptoms in patients < 65 years of age
  - 2. Side effects: somnolence, dizziness, hallucinations, edema, pathologic gambling (impulse control disorders)
- C. MAO-B inhibitors (e.g. selegiline, rasagiline)
  - 1. Usually used for mild symptoms
- D. Amantadine
  - 1. Alternative for MAO-B inhibitors
  - 2. Side effects: livedo reticularis, ankle edema

Parkinson disease

Etiology
Degeneration of dopaminergic neurons in the substantia nigra (motor inhibition)

Epidemiology
Sex: ♀ = ♂
Peak age: 50–60 years

Cardinal symptoms
T - Tremor (resting)
R - Rigidity
A - Akinesia
P - Postural instability

Common early symptoms
Myalgia and arthralgia
Hyposmia
Depression
Obstipation

Life expectancy
Normal with treatment
Patients often become dependent on care in later stages

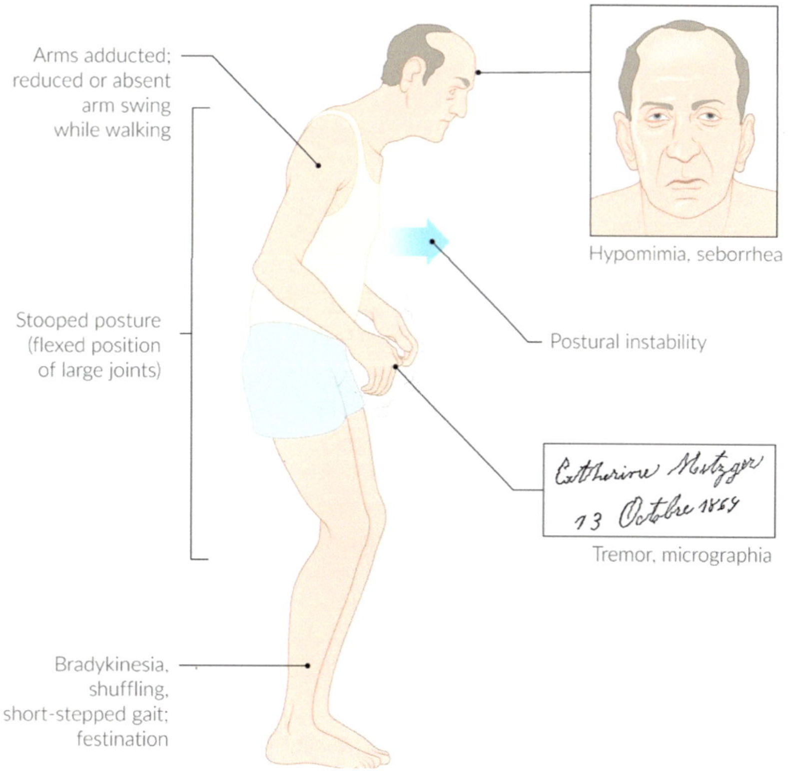

FIGURE 13.1.12 - Parkinson Disease

E. Anticholinergic drugs (e.g. trihexyphenidyl, benztropine)
    1. Young patients with tremor-dominant parkinson disease
    2. Side effects: constipation, dry mouth, urinary retention

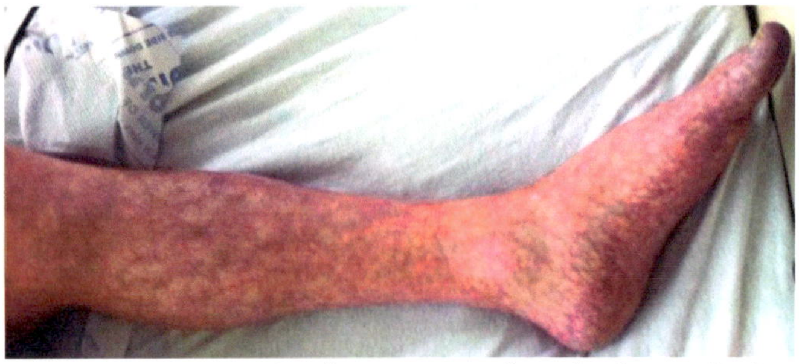

FIGURE 13.1.13 - Livedo Reticularis

V. Huntington Disease: Definition
    A. Inherited neurodegenerative disorder
    B. Autosomal dominant
    C. CAG trinucleotide repeat sequences in HTT gene on chromosome 4
    D. Loss of GABA-producing neurons in neostriatum

VI. Huntington Disease: Clinical Features
    A. Gradual onset of symptoms at 30-50 years of age
    B. Chorea: purposeless, brief, involuntary movements that involve trunk, limbs, and face
    C. Psychiatric disturbances: irritability, depression, antisocial behavior
    D. Dementia
    E. Weight loss & cachexia

VII. Huntington Disease: Diagnosis
    A. Presence of family history and typical clinical findings
    B. Neuroimaging (e.g. MRI): caudate nucleus and putamen atrophy
    C. Genetic testing is confirmatory

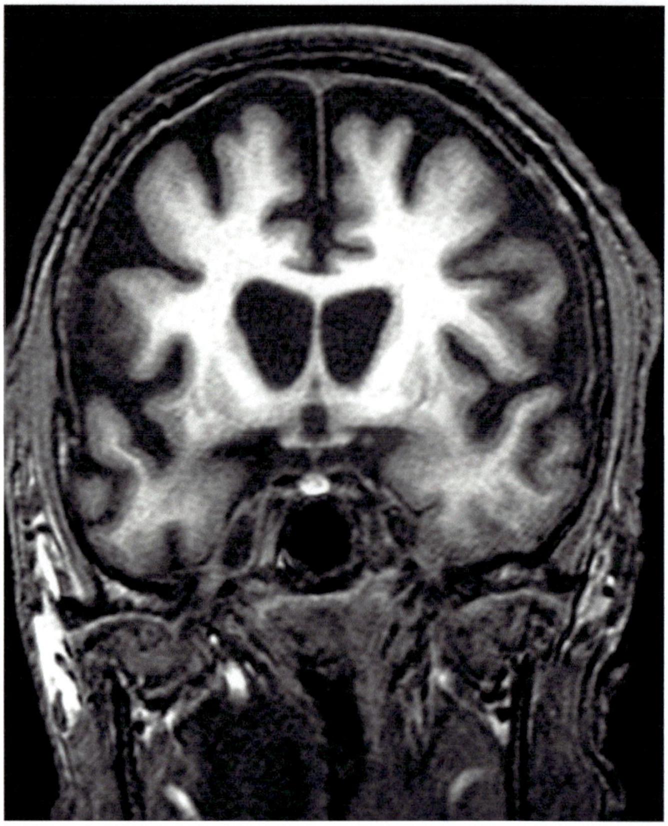

FIGURE 13.1.14 - MRI of Brain: Atrophy of Caudate Nucleus

VIII. Huntington Disease: Management
    A. Treatment is supportive and symptomatic
    B. Survival: 10-20 years after onset

REVIEW QUESTIONS

1. A 67-year-old man is brought to the physician by his wife due to recent behavioral changes in the past 2 weeks. Three years ago the patient started having pill-rolling tremor at rest, a shuffling gait, and stooped posture. One month ago he started having memory problems, he cannot recall the name of his wife and sons. He is experiencing visual hallucinations and sees small creatures running around the house when there is nobody there except his wife. How can this patient's condition be differentiated from Lewy body dementia?
    - **Time between motor and cognitive symptoms is more than 1 year in Parkinson's disease, but less than 1 year in Lewy body dementia.**
    - Three years ago this patient started having pill-rolling tremor at rest, shuffling gait, and stooped posture.
    - One month ago the patient started having memory problems. He cannot recall the name of his family members, and he has visual hallucinations.
    - This description is consistent with Parkinson's disease.
    - Since the time between the motor and cognitive symptoms is more than 1 year, his cognitive decline will be called dementia secondary to Parkinson's disease.

REVIEW QUESTIONS

2. A 45-year-old man is brought to the physician by his wife due to behavioral changes for the last 2 weeks. He has become very aggressive towards his wife and son. He seems depressed with a flat affect. The physical examination shows writhing, slow finger movements and occasional purposeless arm swings. The patient's father suffered from similar symptoms. Based on the patient's fathers condition, what can be assumed about the onset and severity of the patient's condition?

- **More severe and earlier onset of this condition would be expected in the patient's son.**
- This patient is aggressive and depressed with a flat affect.
- The physical exam finding of writhing, slow finger movements is consistent with athetosis. Also, occasional purposeless arm swings suggest chorea.
- His father suffered from similar symptoms.
- Therefore, this patient most likely has Huntington's disease.
- Huntington's disease, just like most of the other trinucleotide repeat disorders, is characterized by anticipation.
- Anticipation means the earlier onset of more severe disease in the patient's offspring due to triplet expansion during gametogenesis.

3. A 62-year-old man comes to the physician because of the worsening of his voluntary movements for the last 3 weeks. He was diagnosed with a neurodegenerative disorder 5 years ago which is controlled with medication. He reports episodes of complete immobility as if he is frozen, followed by episodes of improved mobility. Vital signs include temperature of 37° C (98.6° F), blood pressure of 145/90 mmHg, heart rate of 85 beats/mins, and respiratory rate of 15 breaths/min. The physical exam shows bilateral hand tremor at rest, a narrow, shuffling gait, and an expressionless face. What medication is most likely responsible for this patient's current symptoms?

   A. Levodopa/carbidopa
   B. Amantadine
   C. Ropinirole
   D. Benztropine

- **The correct answer is option A.**
- This patient reports recent worsening of his voluntary movements.
- The physical exam shows bilateral hand tremor at rest, narrow-based and shuffling gait, and expressionless face.
- These findings point towards the diagnosis of Parkinson's disease.
- He reports episodes of complete immobility as if he is frozen, followed by episodes of improved mobility. This description is consistent with the classic "on-off" phenomenon associated with the long-term use of levodopa/carbidopa.
- Option B is incorrect. The main side effects of amantadine include livedo reticularis and ankle edema.
- Option C is incorrect. The side effects of ropinirole include somnolence, dizziness, hallucinations, and impulse control disorders.
- Option D is incorrect. Benztropine is an anticholinergic medication that can cause dry mouth, mydriasis, urinary retention, and constipation.

Neurology | Section 4: Movement Disorders: Tremor & Ataxia

I. Tremor: Definition
   A. Involuntary rhythmic movement involving a part of the body
   B. The most common among movement disorders

II. Tremor: Classification
   A. Rest tremors
      1. Tremor of parkinson disease
   B. Action tremor
      1. Physiologic tremor
      2. Essential tremor (typically familial, AD inheritance)
      3. Cerebellar tremor (e.g. multiple sclerosis, stroke)

III. Tremor: Clinical Features
   A. Tremor of parkinson disease: moderate frequency (4-6 Hz)
      1. Reduced or absent during voluntary movements
      2. Usually involves the hands and legs
      3. May less commonly involve the head
   B. Physiologic tremor: high frequency (12-14 Hz)
      1. Usually undetectable in ordinary conditions
      2. Enhanced by:
         a) Fever, fatigue, anxiety, alcohol withdrawal
         b) Medications: sympathomimetics (e.g. amphetamines, terbutaline), theophyllines, SSRIs, lithium, valproic acid
         c) Metabolic disorders: hyperthyroidism, hypoglycemia
   C. Essential tremor: moderate to high frequency (6-12 Hz)
      1. Typically affects hands and arms, usually bilateral
      2. May affect the head solely
      3. Increased by goal-directed movements (e.g. handwriting, drinking from glass) and outstretching arms
      4. Relieved by alcohol intake
   D. Cerebellar tremor: low frequency (3-4 Hz)
      1. Typically an intention tremor (increases when hand moves toward a target)
      2. May be associated with other cerebellar findings (e.g. ataxia, dysmetria)

IV. Tremor: Diagnosis
   A. Largely dependent on clinical findings, medical history, family history, and physical examination
   B. Laboratory tests: thyroid function tests, electrolytes (e.g. serum calcium)

V. Tremor: Management
   A. Treat the underlying cause or remove the offending factor
   B. Essential tremor:
      1. Beta blockers (first-line): propranolol
      2. Anticonvulsants: primidone

VI. Ataxia: Definition
   A. Uncoordinated movements of the body
   B. May involve limbs or trunk
   C. Can be unilateral or bilateral

VII. Ataxia: Classification
   A. Acquired ataxia
      1. Stroke
      2. Multiple sclerosis
      3. Brain tumor
      4. Vitamin B_{12} deficiency
      5. Alcohol intoxication
   B. Hereditary ataxia
      1. Friedreich ataxia (autosomal recessive)
      2. Ataxia telangiectasia (autosomal recessive)

VIII. Ataxia: Clinical Features
   A. Friedreich ataxia (onset typically in adolescence)
      1. Neurologic features
         a) Progressive cerebellar ataxia
         b) Cerebellar dysarthria
         c) Motor neuropathy, absent DTRs
         d) Loss of proprioception and vibration sense
         e) Hearing loss
      2. Hypertrophic cardiomyopathy (e.g. arrhythmia, heart failure)
      3. Diabetes mellitus
      4. Skeletal features
         a) Kyphoscoliosis, pes cavus, hammer toes, atrophy of intrinsic muscles of hands
   B. Ataxia telangiectasia (onset in childhood)
      1. Progressive cerebellar ataxia
      2. Oculocutaneous telangiectasias
      3. Abnormal eye movements: most common is oculomotor apraxia (uncoordinated head and eye movements when shifting gaze)
      4. Immune deficiency (e.g. recurrent sinopulmonary infections)
      5. Pulmonary disease is the main cause of mortality

Friedreich ataxia

Epidemiology
Incidence: 3–4:100,000
Onset of symptoms: childhood and adolescence (♂ > ♀)

Etiology
Autosomal recessive inheritance:
GAA trinucleotide repeat expansion on chromosom 9 → reduced expression of frataxin protein → disorder of mitochondrial iron metabolism → increased susceptibility to oxidative stress

Complications
Prevalent cause of death: cardiomyopathy

Prognosis
10–15 years after symptom onset most individuals require a wheelchair
Better prognosis with later symptom onset

Life expectancy
Reduced

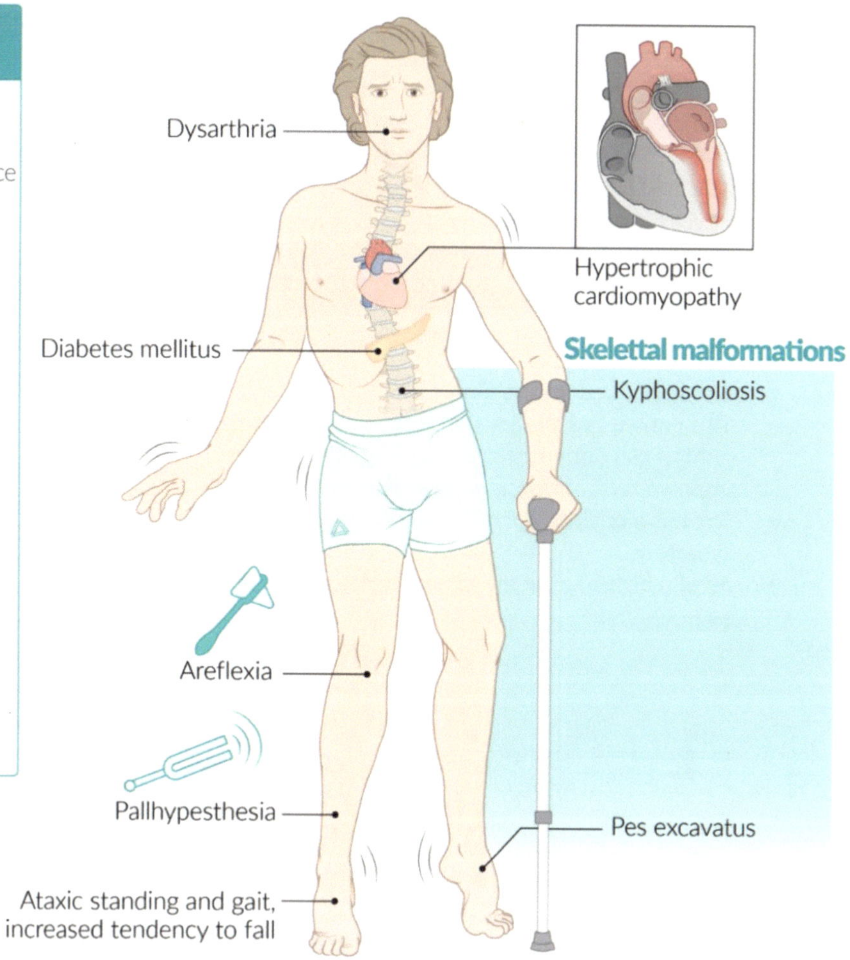

FIGURE 13.1.15 - Friedreich Ataxia

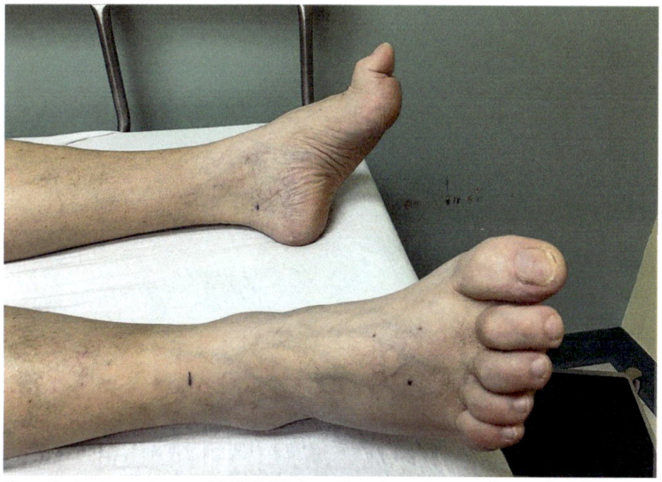

FIGURE 13.1.16 - Hammer Toes

IX. Ataxia: Diagnosis
  A. Friedreich ataxia
    1. Largely based on clinical findings
    2. Genetic testing (confirmatory): expanded trinucleotide GAA repeat in FXN gene on chromosome 9

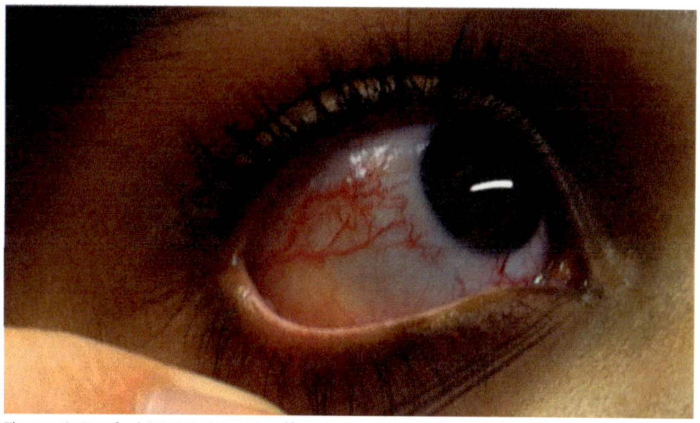

FIGURE 13.1.17 - Conjunctival Telangiectasia

  B. Ataxia telangiectasia
    1. Clinical findings are suggestive
    2. Genetic testing: ATM gene mutation on chromosome 11

X. Ataxia: Management
  A. Friedreich ataxia
    1. No specific therapy
  B. Ataxia telangiectasia
    1. No specific therapy
    2. Median age of mortality is 25 years

REVIEW QUESTIONS

1. A 45-year-old woman comes to her primary care physician because of occasional shaking of both hands for 3-months. She states the shaking worsens when she holds a glass or when she is anxious. Shaking seems to improve after drinking a glass of wine. Her father has similar symptoms. What is the first-line treatment option for this patient's condition?
   - **The first-line treatment for this patient's condition is propranolol.**
   - This patient has tremor that worsens when she holds a glass or when she is anxious. The tremor improves after drinking a glass of wine.
   - She has a positive family history for the similar symptoms.
   - All of which suggest the patient has an essential tremor.

2. A 15-year-old boy is brought to the pediatrician for a follow-up visit. He uses a cane to ambulate. Physical exam shows spastic paralysis of the lower extremities, ataxia, and loss of vibration and proprioception over his entire body. Examination also shows kyphoscoliosis. Laboratory studies show fasting blood glucose of 300 mg/dL (70-100 mg/dL) which has now been consistent on 2 separate occasions. What is the most likely abnormality to be seen on echocardiography of this patient?
   - **The most likely abnormality to be seen on echocardiography of this patient with Friedreich ataxia is hypertrophic cardiomyopathy.**
   - This patient uses the cane to ambulate.
   - The physical examination shows spastic paralysis of lower extremities, likely due to degeneration of lateral corticospinal tracts; ataxia likely caused by damage to spinocerebellar tract; and loss of vibration and proprioception that can be explained by degeneration of dorsal columns. He also has kyphoscoliosis.
   - He has diabetes mellitus based on his fasting blood glucose levels.
   - All of these findings suggest the diagnosis of Friedreich ataxia.

Neurology | Section 5: Movement Disorders: Restless Leg Syndrome & Tourette Syndrome

I. Restless Leg Syndrome: Definition
   A. Sleep-related movement disorder
   B. May be primary (idiopathic) or secondary (associated with comorbid condition)

II. Restless Leg Syndrome: Risk Factors
   A. Family history
   B. Iron deficiency anemia
   C. Uremia
   D. Pregnancy
   E. Multiple sclerosis, Parkinson disease, neuropathy
   F. Medications (e.g. metoclopramide)

III. Restless Leg Syndrome: Clinical Features
   A. Unpleasant urge to move the legs
      1. Feels like "crawling", "tension", "electric", "creeping", "itching"
   B. Most commonly in evening and at rest
   C. Typically relieved by movement (e.g. walking, stretching)

IV. Restless Leg Syndrome: Diagnosis
   A. Diagnostic criteria
      1. Urge to move the legs, usually with uncomfortable sensations
      2. Symptoms begin/worsen during rest or inactivity
      3. Symptoms are worse in evening or night
      4. Symptoms partially or totally relieved by movement
      5. Symptoms cannot be explained by another condition

V. Restless Leg Syndrome: Management
   A. Oral iron therapy if serum ferritin < 75 mcg/L
   B. Mild symptoms: avoiding aggravating factors, exercise, leg massage
   C. Moderate/severe or persistent symptoms
      1. Dopamine agonists (e.g. pramipexole)
      2. Alpha-2-delta calcium channel ligand (e.g. gabapentin)

VI. Tourette Syndrome: Definition
   A. Chronic neurologic disorder
   B. Motor and phonic tics
   C. Genetic predisposition

VII. Tourette Syndrome: Clinical Features
   A. Tics: sudden, brief, intermittent movements/sounds
      1. Onset is 2-15 years of age
      2. Motor tics: blinking, facial grimace, shoulder shrugging, copropraxia, echopraxia
      3. Phonic tics: moaning, sniffing, grunting, coprolalia, echolalia
      4. Symptoms improve during adolescence and adulthood
   B. Comorbidities
      1. Attention deficit hyperactivity disorder
      2. Obsessive compulsive disorder

VIII. Tourette Syndrome: Diagnosis
   A. Diagnostic criteria
      1. Multiple motor tics and ≥ 1 phonic tics
      2. Tics are recurrent (multiple times a day, nearly every day)
      3. Tics last > 1 year
      4. Onset before 18 years of age
      5. Tics cannot be explained by other conditions

IX. Tourette Syndrome: Management
   A. Comprehensive Behavioral Intervention for Tics (CBIT)
   B. Medications: tetrabenazine
   C. Botulinum toxin injections

REVIEW QUESTIONS

1. A 60-year-old man comes to the clinic because of a crawling sensation over his legs when he lies down in bed at night for the past month. The crawling sensation improves when he massages his legs or walks around the bed. His wife has recently complained of him "kicking his legs in sleep." Colonoscopy 10-years ago revealed several hyperplastic polyps in his sigmoid colon. Serum creatinine and BUN are normal. Which laboratory test should be ordered next to help determine the cause of this patient's symptoms?

- **An iron panel: serum ferritin, serum iron, total iron binding capacity, and transferrin saturation should be ordered for this patient.**
- This patient has a crawling sensation over his legs when he lies down in bed at night. This sensation improves when he massages his legs or walks around the bed. He also has involuntary leg movements at night.
- All these findings point towards the diagnosis of restless leg syndrome.
- Restless leg syndrome is commonly associated with chronic kidney disease and iron deficiency anemia.
- His serum creatinine and BUN are normal making chronic kidney disease unlikely.
- Considering that he has hyperplastic polyps in the sigmoid colon, he may have occult gastrointestinal bleeding and resultant iron deficiency anemia triggering the restless leg syndrome.

2. A 9-year-old boy is brought to the pediatrician by his parents because of difficulties at school for the past year. His classmates make fun of him because he makes grunting and barking sounds during class. His parents have also noticed occasional head thrusts, eye blinks, and facial grimacing at home. Vital signs are unremarkable. Throughout the examination the patient makes intermittent eye blinks and a barking sound. Parents ask about the prognosis of their son's condition. Which of the following conditions is this patient at risk to develop?

A. Oppositional defiant disorder
B. Attention deficit hyperactivity disorder
C. Disruptive mood dysregulation disorder
D. Autism spectrum disorder

- **The correct answer is option B.**
- This 9-year-old boy has been making grunting and barking sounds for the past year. These are considered to be vocal tics.
- The parents have also noticed occasional head thrusts, eye blinks, and facial grimacing at home. Therefore, the patient also has multiple motor tics.
- Multiple vocal and motor tics lasting at least a year in a person less than 18 years of age are consistent with the diagnosis of Tourette syndrome.
- Tourette syndrome is mainly associated with two comorbidities: obsessive-compulsive disorder and attention deficit hyperactivity disorder. Therefore, this patient is at risk for developing attention deficit hyperactivity disorder.
- Option A, oppositional defiant disorder, option C, disruptive mood dysregulation disorder, and option D, autism spectrum disorder, are incorrect because these conditions are not associated with Tourette syndrome.

Neurology | Section 6: Meningitis

I. Meningitis: Definition
   A. Inflammation of leptomeninges that surround the brain and spinal cord

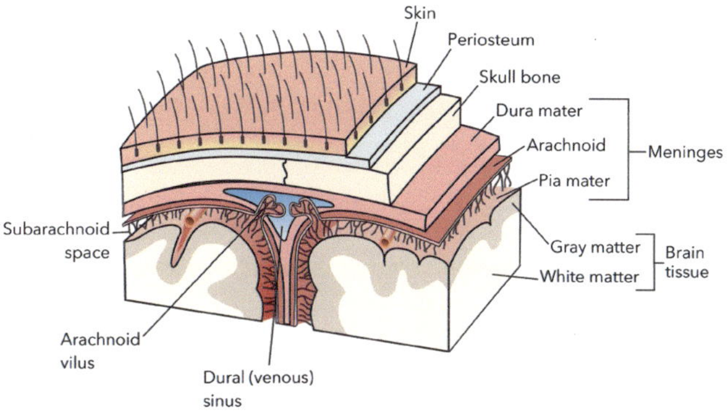

FIGURE 13.1.18 - Meninges

II. Meningitis: Etiology
   A. Bacterial
      1. *S. pneumoniae* (most common pathogen of community-acquired bacterial meningitis)
      2. *N. meningitidis* (most common in children and young adults)
      3. *H. influenza*
      4. *Listeria*
   B. Mycobacterial (e.g. *M. tuberculosis*)
   C. Viral (e.g. enteroviruses)
   D. Fungal (e.g. *Cryptococcus neoformans*)

III. Meningitis: Clinical Features
   A. Classic triad: fever, nuchal rigidity, mental status changes
   B. Headache, nausea, vomiting, photophobia
   C. Physical examination: kernig, brudzinski

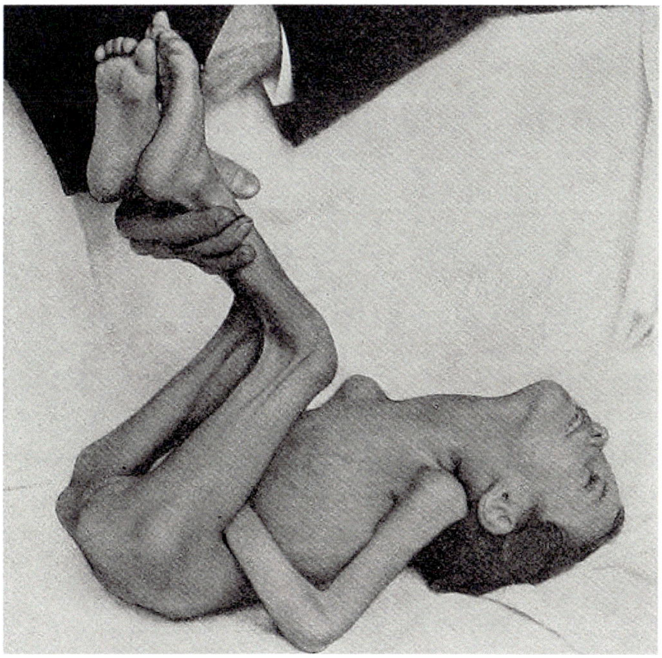

FIGURE 13.1.19 - Kernig Sign

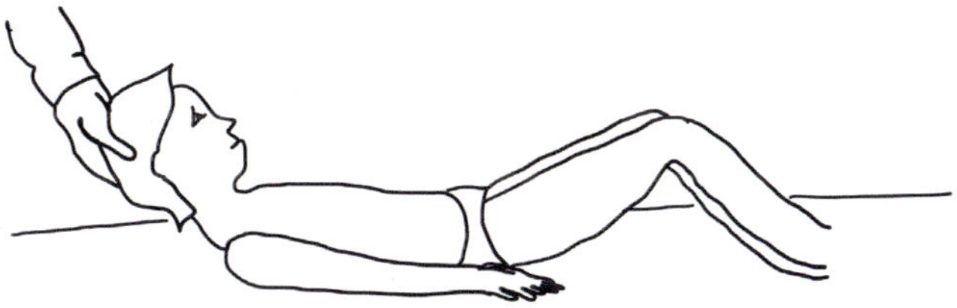

FIGURE 13.1.20 - Brudzinski Sign

IV. Meningococcal Meningitis
   A. Pathogen: *Neisseria meningitidis*
   B. Acute onset
   C. Severe myalgias, non-suppurative pharyngitis, rapidly progressive illness
   D. Physical examination: petechial/hemorrhagic rash, pale and mottled skin
   E. Complications: shock, DIC, Waterhouse-Friderichsen syndrome

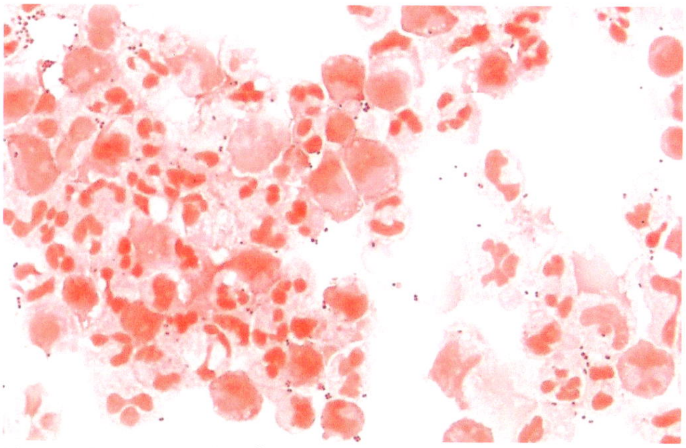

FIGURE 13.1.21 - Light Microscopy of Gram Stained CSF Sample: Gram-Negative Diplococci

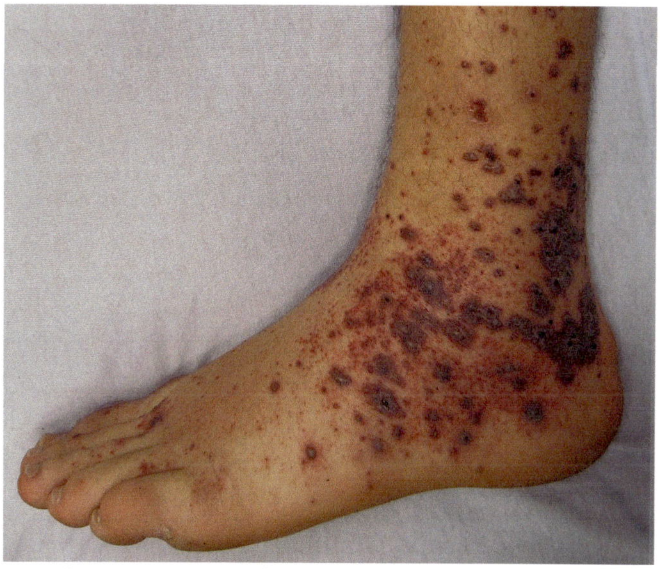

FIGURE 13.1.22 - Petechiae and Purpura

V. Cryptococcal Meningoencephalitis
   A. Opportunistic infection by *Cryptococcus neoformans*
   B. Most commonly affects HIV patients with CD4 < 100/microL
   C. Subacute onset (over 1-2 weeks)
      1. Fever, headache, malaise
      2. Signs of elevated ICP (e.g. papilledema, CN VI deficit)
      3. Photophobia and nuchal rigidity are usually absent
   D. Umbilicated skin lesions can be seen (disseminated disease)

VI. Tuberculous Meningitis
   A. Pathogen: *Mycobacterium tuberculosis*
   B. Subacute onset
      1. Headache, fever, nuchal rigidity
      2. Confusion, CN palsies (most commonly II & VI), seizures and coma in late stages
   C. Hydrocephalus is a common complication due to obstruction of basilar cisterns (signs of ↑ ICP)

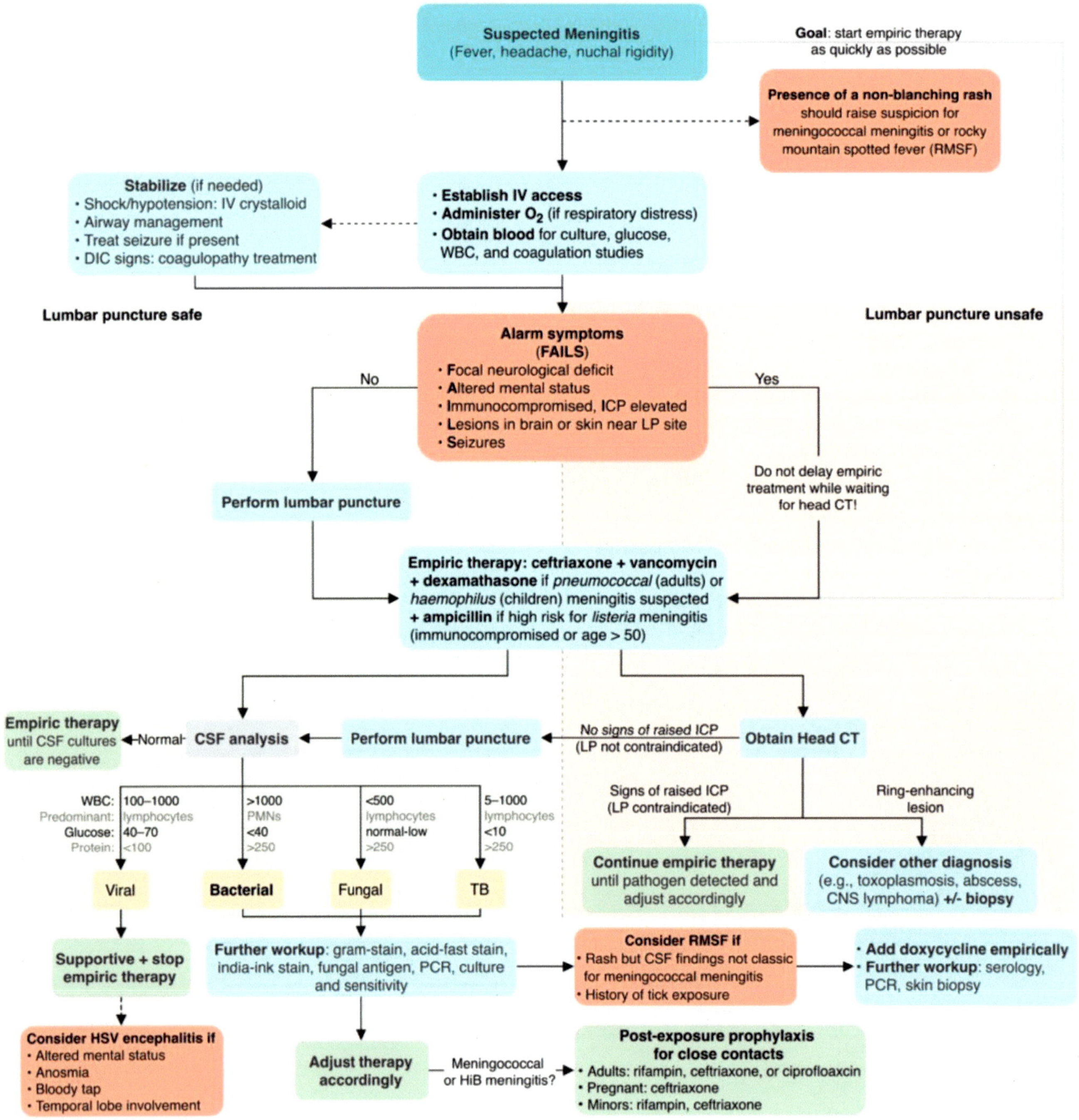

FIGURE 13.1.26 - Diagnosis and Management of Meningitis

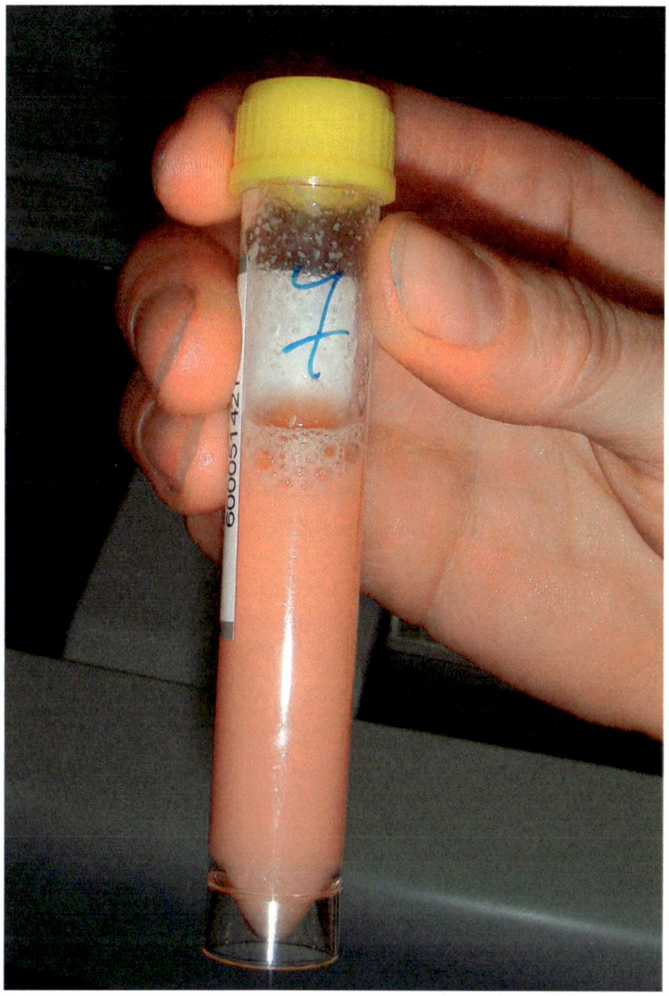

FIGURE 13.1.27 - Purulent CSF Sample

REVIEW QUESTIONS

1. A 35-year-old female is rushed to the emergency department via ambulance due to the sudden onset of altered mental status. In the emergency department she was found to be hypotensive. Laboratory studies show hyponatremia, hyperkalemia, hypoglycemia, as well as metabolic acidosis. The patient's husband shtates she had been experiencing a fever and neck stiffness over the last few days. Which organism is most likely responsible for this patient's condition?
    - ***Neisseria meningitidis*, a Gram-negative diplococci, is most likely responsible for this patient's condition.**
    - This patient presents with sudden onset hypotension, hyponatremia, hyperkalemia, hypoglycemia, and metabolic acidosis.
    - This constellation of features should suggest an acute adrenal crisis.
    - The patient has also experienced fever and neck stiffness which, along with mental status changes if present, make up the classic triad of meningitis.
    - An acute adrenal crisis, brought on by a serious bacterial infection, is known as Waterhouse-Friderichsen syndrome which is most commonly caused by disseminated *Neisseria meningitidis* infections.

Neurology | Section 7: Encephalitis

I. Encephalitis: Definition
   A. Inflammation of brain parenchyma
   B. Usually of viral etiology (e.g. HSV, West Nile virus)

II. Encephalitis: Clinical Features
   A. Fever, headache, nausea
   B. Altered mental status (e.g. confusion, agitation)
   C. Neurologic deficits (e.g. hemiparesis, focal CN deficits, aphasia, hyperreflexia)
   D. Seizures

III. Encephalitis: Diagnosis
   A. CT (to exclude space-occupying lesion prior to LP)
   B. Lumbar puncture and CSF analysis
   C. MRI
   D. Electroencephalography
   E. CSF PCR
   F. Serologic testing (e.g. IgM antibodies for West Nile virus in CSF)

IV. HSV Encephalitis
   A. HSV should be the first pathogen to exclude in encephalitis
   B. Acute onset
   C. Behavioral syndromes can be seen (e.g. Klüver-Bucy syndrome, hypomania)
   D. CSF analysis: ↑ red blood cell count
   E. MRI: abnormal signal in temporal lobes
   F. CSF PCR is the gold standard to confirm diagnosis

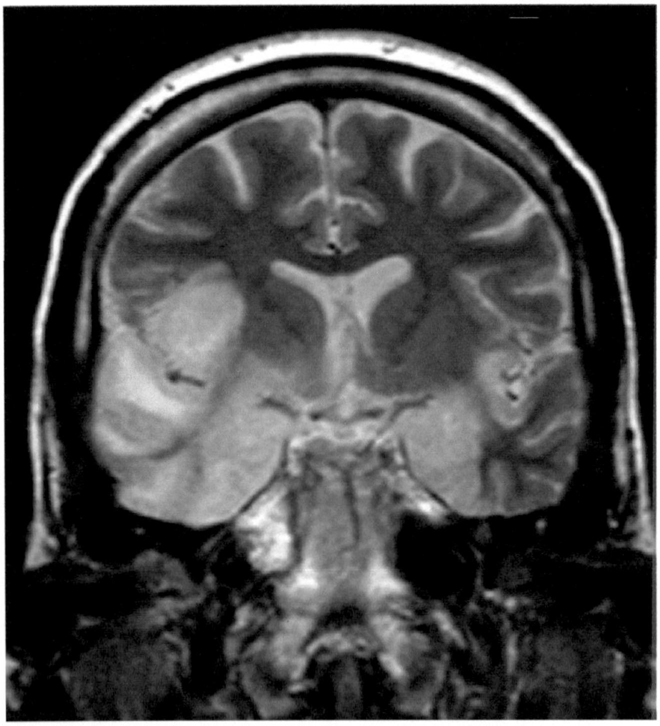

FIGURE 13.1.28 - MRI of the Brain: Temporal Lobe Hyperintensity in HSV Encephalitis

V. *Toxoplasma* Encephalitis
   A. Reactivation of *Toxoplasma gondii* from prior infection
   B. Most common manifestation of toxoplasmosis
   C. Typically affects HIV patients with CD4 < 100/microL
   D. Multiple ring-enhancing lesions on MRI
   E. Serologic testing: positive *Toxoplasma gondii* IgG antibodies

VI. Encephalitis: Management
   A. Empiric therapy: IV acyclovir
   B. Supportive therapy
   C. Toxoplasma encephalitis: sulfadiazine & pyrimethamine + leucovorin

REVIEW QUESTIONS

1. A 65-year-old man is brought to the emergency room via ambulance after having a witnessed seizure at work 30-minutes ago. On arrival he is confused and states he has a "horrible headache". Vitals signs are notable for a temperature of 102.4F. The patient's spouse arrives and mentions that the patient has recently been behaving out of character. MRI of the brain and brainstem is performed and shows bi-temporal hyperintensities. What is the best next step in management for this patient?

   - **The next best step in management is immediate initiation IV acyclovir.**
   - The patient presents following a seizure, and per his spouse has a recent change in personality.
   - MRI of the brain shows bi-temporal hyperintensities, highly suggestive for HSV encephalitis.
   - With such a high suspicion for HSV encephalitis initiation of treatment should not be postponed while completing the work-up.
   - After initiation of IV acyclovir, lumbar punctures should be performed and CSF sent for analysis.

Neurology | Section 8: Brain Abscess & Spinal Epidural Abscess

I. Brain Abscess: Definition
   A. Focal collection of pus in the brain
   B. Develops as complication of infection or trauma
   C. Most common pathogens are *Streptococcus viridans* and *Staphylococcus aureus*

II. Brain Abscess: Pathophysiology
   A. Bacteria reaches brain parenchyma through:
      1. Direct spread from contagious site (typically single abscess)
         a) Otitis media, mastoiditis (temporal lobe)
         b) Frontal or ethmoidal sinusitis (frontal lobe)
      2. Hematogenous spread (typically multiple abscesses)
         a) Bacterial endocarditis, skin and soft tissue infections
      3. Neurosurgery/penetrating trauma

III. Brain Abscess: Pathology
   A. Early lesion (cerebritis): first 1-2 weeks
      1. Acute inflammation with localized edema, no necrosis
      2. Infiltration of neutrophils
   B. Late lesion
      1. Central necrosis, formation of fibrotic capsule
      2. Infiltration of macrophages

IV. Brain Abscess: Clinical Features
   A. Severe headache (most common): usually unilateral and resistant to analgesics
   B. Focal neurologic deficits
   C. Seizures

V. Brain Abscess: Diagnosis
   A. CT (emergent situations)
   B. MRI (imaging study of choice)
   C. Brain biopsy (accurately defines causative pathogen)

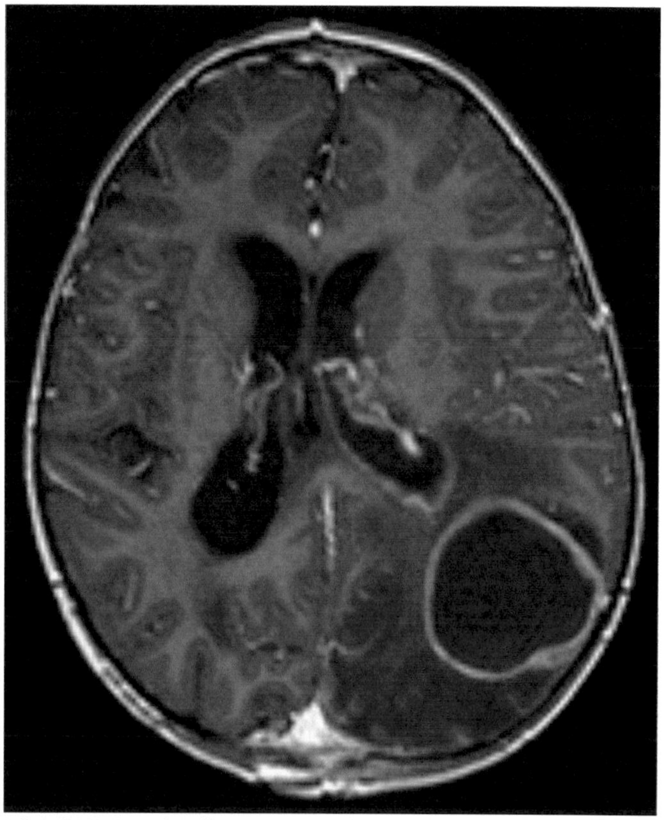

FIGURE 13.1.29 - MRI of the Brain: Brain Abscess

VI. Brain Abscess: Management
   A. IV empiric therapy (immediately after diagnostic aspiration/biopsy)
      1. Oral/otogenic/sinus source of infection: metronidazole + ceftriaxone/cefotaxime
      2. Hematogenous spread: vancomycin
      3. Penetrating trauma: vancomycin + ceftriaxone/cefotaxime
   B. Tailoring therapy (4-8 weeks)
   C. Surgery: needle aspiration, surgical excision

VII. Spinal Epidural Abscess: Definition
   A. Suppurative infection that forms in the space between vertebral wall and dura mater of spinal cord
   B. Most common pathogen is *Staphylococcus aureus*

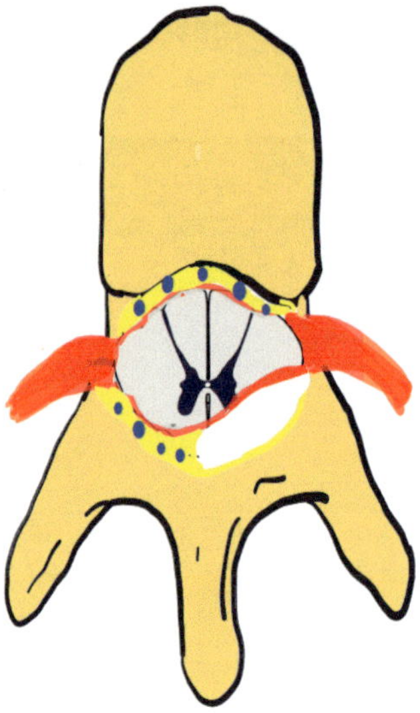

FIGURE 13.1.30 - Spinal Epidural Abscess

VIII. Spinal Epidural Abscess: Pathophysiology

A. Bacteria enters epidural space by:
   1. Hematogenous spread (e.g. cellulitis, bacterial endocarditis, injection drug use)
   2. Direct extension from contagious tissues (e.g. vertebral osteomyelitis)
   3. Inoculation into spinal canal (e.g. epidural catheters)

IX. Spinal Epidural Abscess: Risk Factors

A. Injection drug use
B. Infective endocarditis
C. Dental abscess
D. Spinal or epidural procedure
E. Immunocompromised states (e.g. HIV infection, diabetes mellitus, alcoholism)

X. Spinal Epidural Abscess: Clinical Features

A. Classic triad
   1. Fever
   2. Focal back pain
   3. Progressive neurologic deficits (e.g. sensory and motor deficits, bladder dysfunction)

XI. Spinal Epidural Abscess: Diagnosis

A. Elevated ESR & CRP
B. Imaging studies: MRI with contrast (imaging study of choice), CT with contrast
C. Blood cultures
D. Abscess specimens

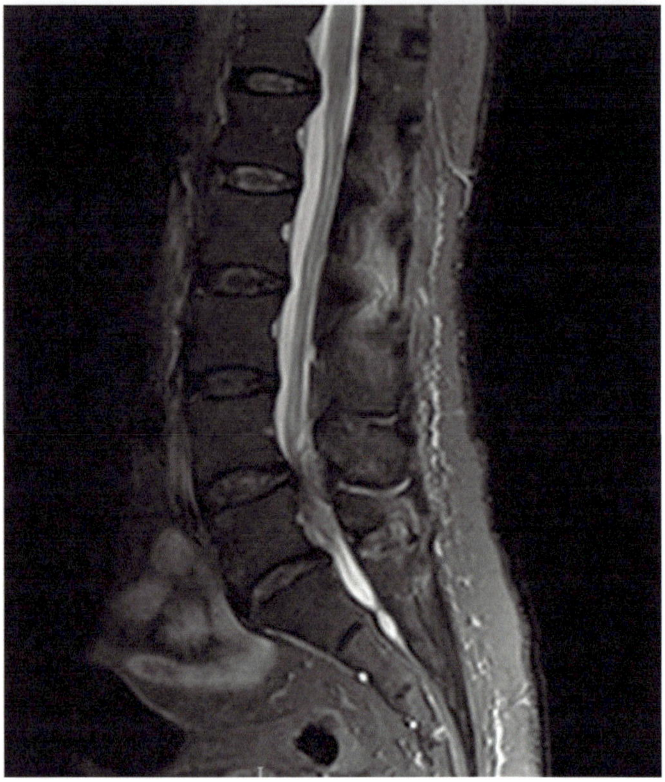

FIGURE 13.1.31 - MRI of the Spinal Cord: Spinal Epidural Abscess

XII. Spinal Epidural Abscess: Management

A. Empiric antibiotics (immediately after obtaining blood)
   1. Vancomycin + 3rd or 4th-generation cephalosporin
B. Tailoring therapy
C. Surgical drainage and decompression (progressive neurological deficits, ring-enhancing lesions on MRI, spinal instability, progression of disease despite antimicrobial therapy

REVIEW QUESTIONS

1. A patient recently presented to the emergency room because of altered mental studies. Emergent CT scan without contrast is performed and shows multiple brain abscesses. What is the most likely route taken by the organism to spread to the brain?

    - **This patient's imaging shows multiple abscesses, therefore a hematogenous route would be suspected.**
    - There are three main routes bacteria can take to enter the brain parenchyma: direct spread, hematogenous spread, and neurosurgery or penetrating trauma.
    - Looking at only brain scans, a surgical or traumatic insult would be obvious with disruption of the normal brain parenchyma.
    - Direct spread and hematogenous spread can be differentiated by the number of abscesses.
    - Direct spread from a site near the brain typically presents as single abscess relatively near the original site, while hematogenous spread from distal sites typically presents as multiple abscesses since the bacteria is carried by the blood and it can theoretically end up anywhere in the brain near a vascular supply.

2. A 68-year-old man comes to the emergency department because of a severe right-sided headache accompanied by ear pain for 3-day. Vitals are significant for a temperature of 101.2° F (38.4° C). He notes that he took 1g of Tylenol which did not help at all. Physical exam shows a swollen and tender mastoid process. He is diagnosed with mastoiditis and imaging ultimately reveals a single brain abscess. Which of the following is the best treatment regimen?

    A. Fluconazole + cefotaxime
    B. Metronidazole + ceftriaxone
    C. Vancomycin
    D. Vancomycin + ceftriaxone

    - **The correct answer is option B.**
    - This 68-year-old-man presents complaining of a severe right sided headache, ear pain, and fever which has not improved by over the counter analgesics.
    - Physical examination shows a swollen tender mastoid process.
    - Imagining reveals a brain abscess likely caused by direct spread of bacteria from the patient's mastoiditis.
    - The empiric therapy for brain abscesses differs based on the bacterial route of entry into the brain parenchyma.
    - In this case, the bacteria has likely spread to the brain from the mastoid, and therefore should be treated with metronidazole + ceftriaxone or cefotaxime.
    - Option A is incorrect because fluconazole is an antifungal medication which is not indicated in bacterial infections.
    - Option C is incorrect because vancomycin alone is used to treat brain abscesses which occurs in the setting of hematogenous spread of bacteria to the brain.
    - Option D is incorrect because vancomycin + ceftriaxone is used to treat brain abscesses which occurs in the setting of penetrating trauma allowing bacteria to enter the brain.

Neurology | Section 9: Dementia

I. Dementia: General Characteristics
   A. Common cause of declining intellectual and cognitive function and mortality in the elderly
   B. Impairment in memory, orientation, visuospatial skills, language and executive functions (e.g. planning and activities of daily living)
   C. Preservation of consciousness
   D. Major risk factor is increasing age

II. Dementia: Differential Diagnosis
   A. Alzheimer disease
      1. Slow onset, early short-term memory loss
      2. Language problems, difficulty with ADLs, spatial disorientation
      3. Later personality changes
   B. Vascular dementia
      1. Stepwise decline, executive dysfunction
      2. Cerebral infarction, deep white matter changes
   C. Frontotemporal dementia (Pick's disease)
      1. Early personality changes, disinhibition, apathy
      2. Compulsive and inappropriate behavior, language problems
      3. Frontotemporal atrophy
   D. Dementia with lewy bodies
      1. Visual hallucinations, REM sleep behavior disorder
      2. Fluctuating cognition, parkinsonism
   E. Normal pressure hydrocephalus
      1. Ataxia, urinary incontinence, dementia
      2. Dilated ventricles on imaging
   F. Prion disease
      1. Rapid progression
      2. Startle myoclonus, seizures
      3. Behavioral changes
   G. Korsakoff dementia
      1. Thiamine deficiency, damaged mammillary bodies
      2. Amnesia, confabulation
      3. Lack of insight
      4. Apathy
      5. Impaired executive functioning

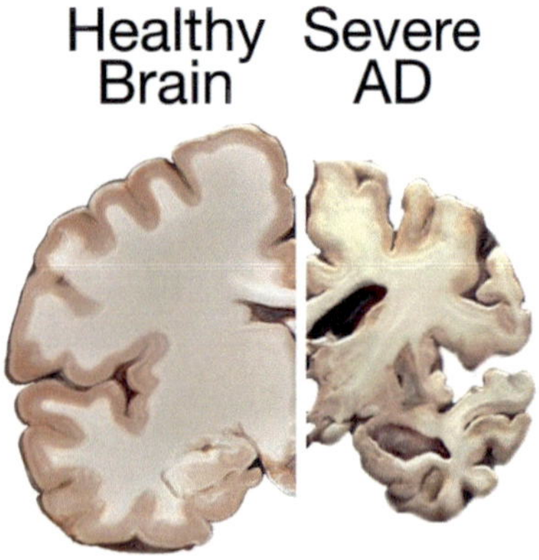

FIGURE 13.1.32 - Healthy Brain vs. Brain in Severe Alzheimer's Dementia

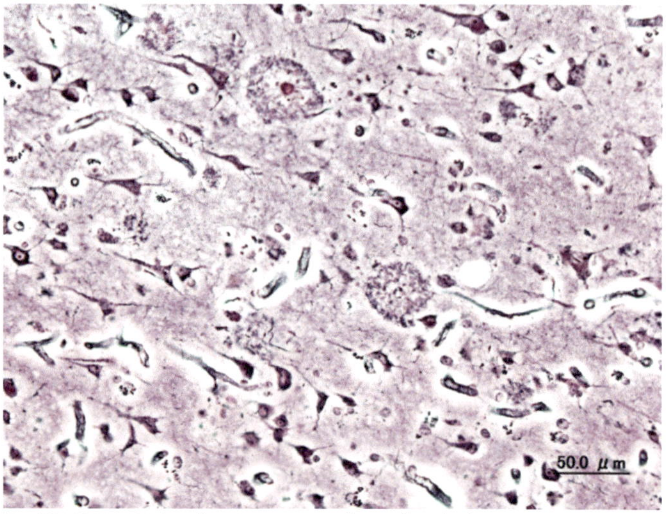

FIGURE 13.1.33 - Light Microscopy: Senile Plaques in Alzheimer's Dementia

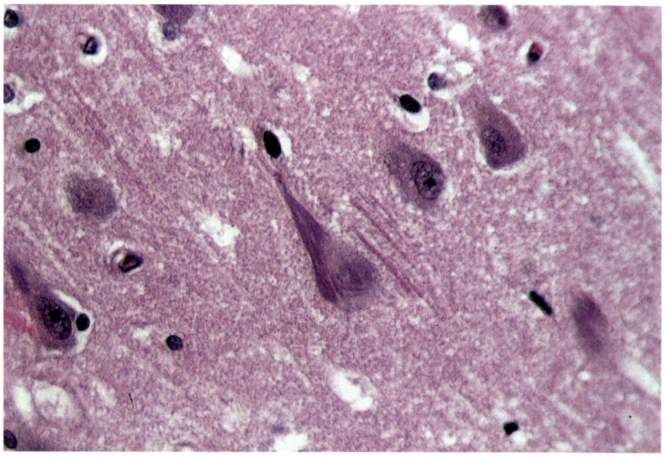

FIGURE 13.1.34 - Light Microscopy: Neurofibrillary Tangles in Alzheimer's Dementia

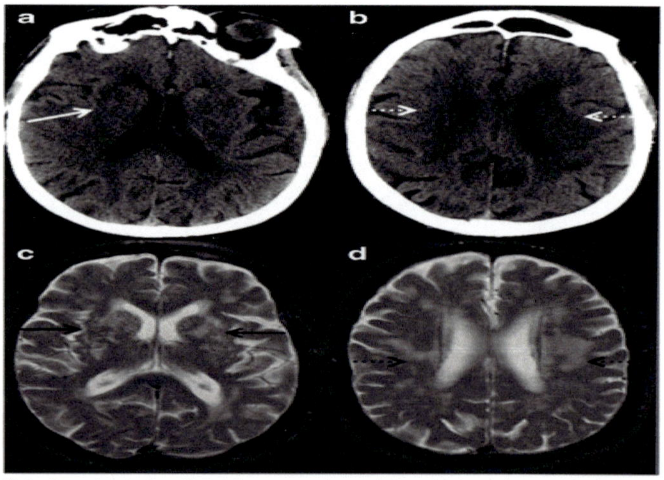

FIGURE 13.1.35 - CT Scan of the Brain: Multiple Hypodensities in Periventricular and Subcortical White Matter and Basal Ganglia in Vascular Dementia

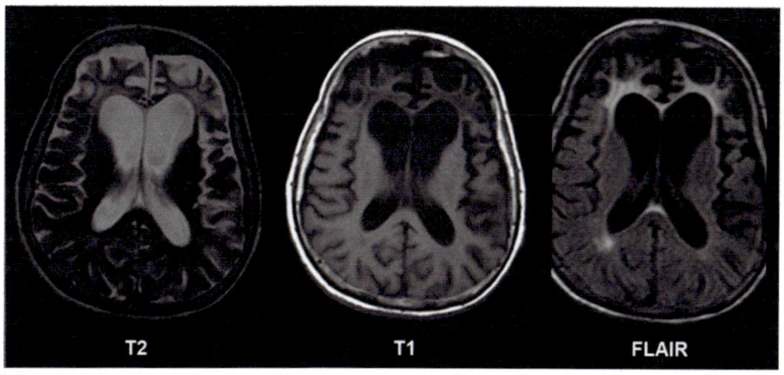

FIGURE 31.1.36 - MRI of the Brain: Atrophy of Frontal and Temporal Lobes in Frontotemporal Dementia

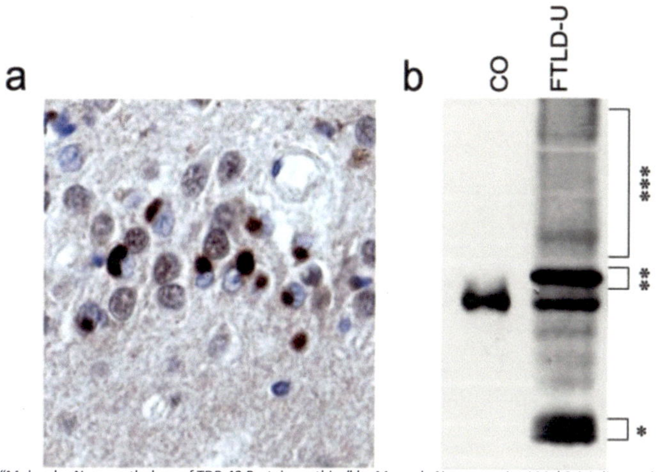

FIGURE 13.1.37 - Light Microscopy: Pick Bodies

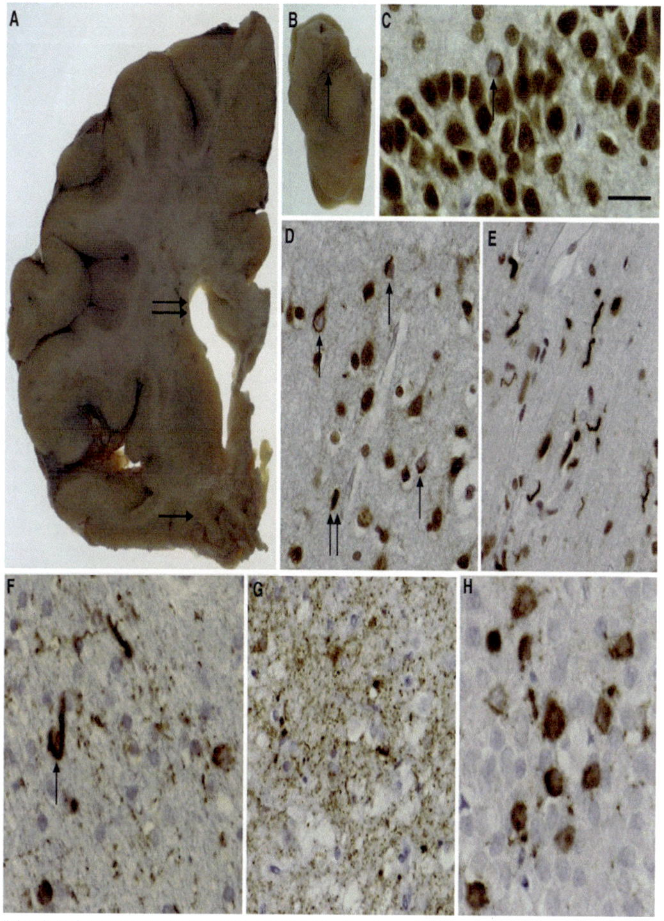

FIGURE 13.1.38 - Enlarged Ventricles and Atrophy of Temporal Lobe in Frontotemporal Dementia

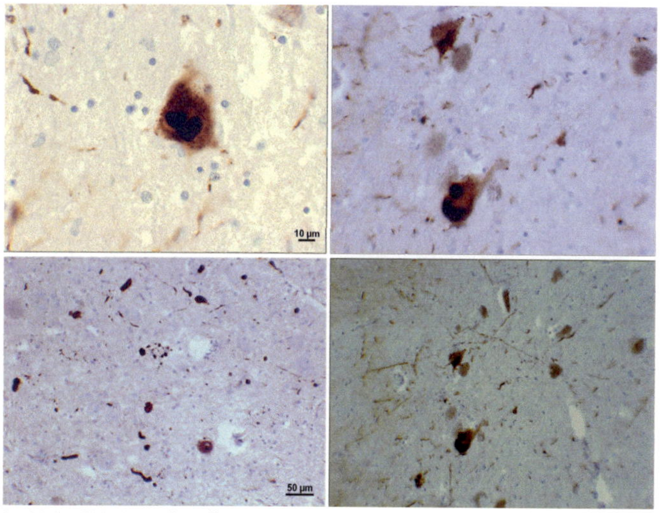

FIGURE 13.1.39 - Light Microscopy: Lewy Body

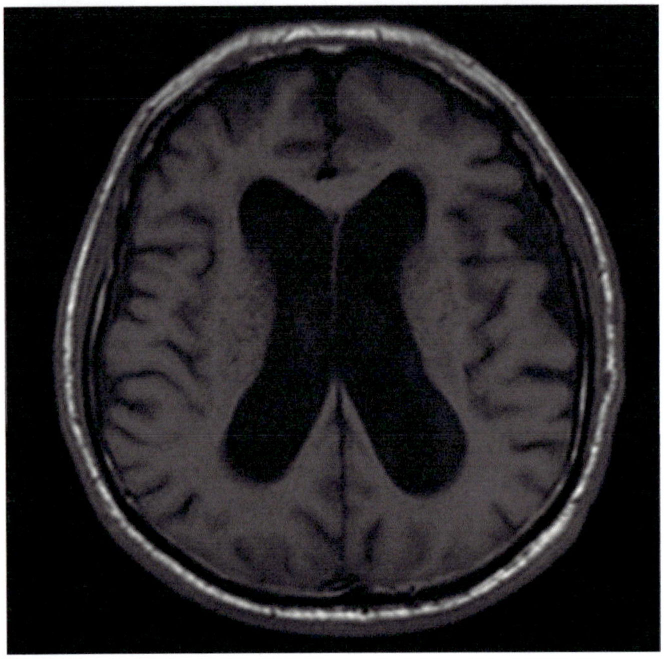

FIGURE 13.1.40 - MRI of the Brain: Enlarged Ventricles in Normal Pressure Hydrocephalus

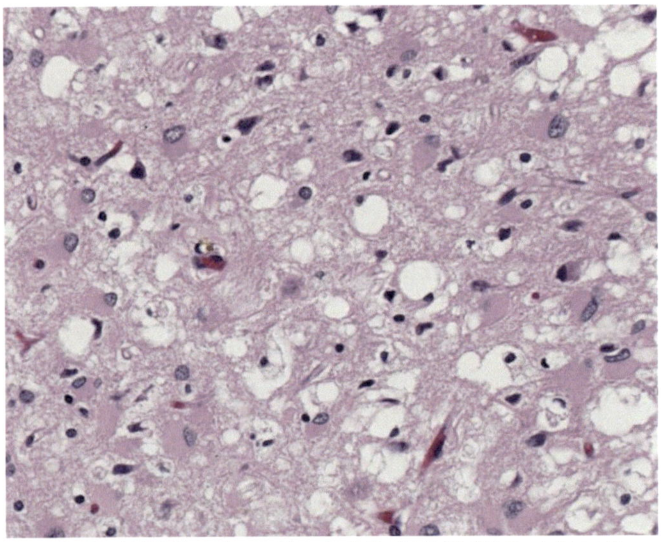

FIGURE 13.1.41 - Light Microscopy: Spongiform Changes in Creutzfeldt-Jakob Disease

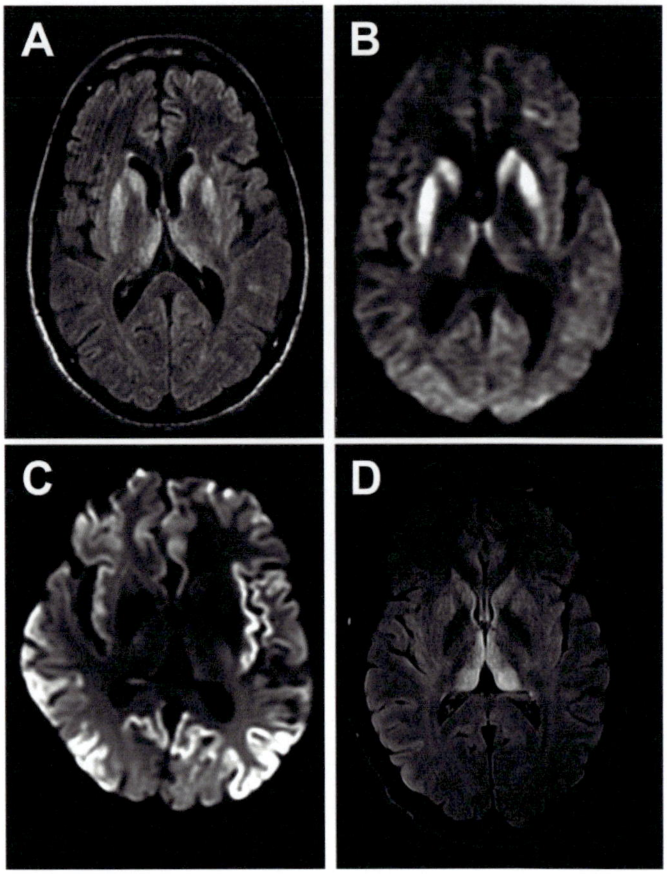

FIGURE 13.1.42 - MRI of the Brain: Hyperintense Signals in the Cortex and Basal Ganglia in Creutzfeldt-Jakob Disease

III. Dementia: Clinical Approach
    A. Routine laboratory tests
        1. CBC, TSH, B_{12}
        2. Selective tests (e.g. folate, VDRL)
    B. Depression screening
    C. Mini mental state exam
    D. Imaging
        1. CT or MRI

MINI MENTAL STATE EXAMINATION

Orientation Name, location, date, present fact.	
Registration Examiner names 3 objects and asks the patient to repeat it	
Attention and Calculation Subtract 7 from 100, then, repeat. Continue this five times.	
Recall Ask for the names of the 3 objects learned earlier.	
Language Name two objects Repeat "No ifs, ands, or buts" Give a three-stage command. Score 1 for each stage. Ask the patient to read and obey a written command. Ask the patient to write a sentence.	Scoring 24-30 : no cognitive impairment 18-23 : mild cognitive impairment 0-17 : severe cognitive impairment
Copying Ask the patient to copy a pair of intersecting pentagons	

FIGURE 13.1.43 - Mini Mental State Examination

IV. Dementia: Treatment
   A. Alzheimer disease
      1. Acetylcholinesterase inhibitors (donepezil, rivastigmine, galantamine)
      2. Memantine
   B. Vascular dementia
      1. Lifestyle modifications (e.g. weight loss, low salt, no smoking)
      2. Treat underlying conditions (e.g. DM, HTN, hyperlipidemia)
   C. Frontotemporal dementia (Pick's disease)
      1. Symptomatic treatment (e.g. physical and speech therapy, SSRI, antipsychotics with caution)
   D. Dementia with lewy bodies
      1. Donepezil, rivastigmine, galantamine, memantine
      2. Levodopa, haloperidol
   E. Normal-pressure hydrocephalus
      1. Lumbar puncture, lumbar drain trial
      2. If responsive to LP, place shunt
   F. Korsakoff dementia and disease
      1. Thiamine followed by glucose
   G. Prion disease
      1. No effective treatment

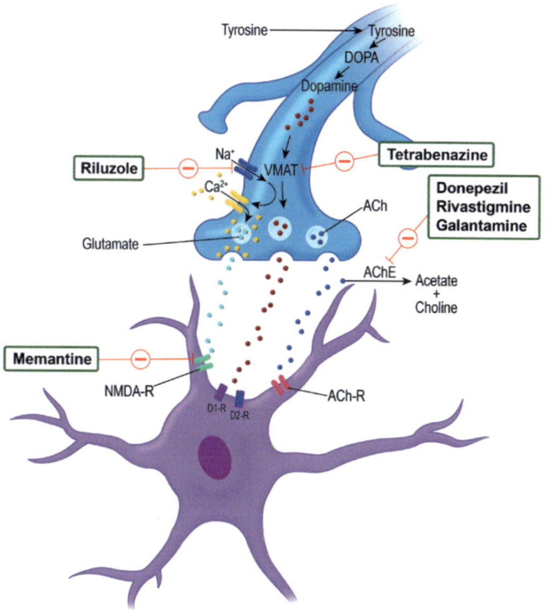

FIGURE 13.1.44 - Mechanism of Action of Certain Medications

REVIEW QUESTIONS

1. A 78-year-old man is brought to the physician by his son due to worsening memory problems for the last 2 years. It began with him misplacing items at home, then getting lost in his neighborhood, and now he has a hard time remembering who he is. He has a history of uncontrolled hypertension and hypercholesterolemia. Physical examination shows right-sided hemiparesis. What is the most likely diagnosis?
   - **The most likely diagnosis is vascular dementia.**
   - This patient presents with worsening memory problems for the last 2 years.
   - In the beginning he would misplace objects at home, then he began getting lost in his neighborhood, and now he has a hard time remembering who he is. These are the signs of stepwise decline in the patient's cognitive functioning.
   - Considering his hypertension and hypercholesterolemia and the presence of the right-sided hemiparesis, this patient likely had at least one episode of stroke.
   - Dementia along with vasculopathy and the focal neurological deficits is consistent with vascular dementia.

2. An 81-year-old woman is brought to the physician by her daughter due to strange behavior for the past 6 months. On some days the patient behaves as usual but on other days, she is irritable and cannot recognize her daughter. She also claims that she sometimes sees two tigers at home. She has a 3 month history of postural instability, shuffling gait, and resting tremor. What sleep disturbance is expected in this patient?
   - **The sleep disorder expected in this patient is REM sleep behavior disorder.**
   - This patient has had strange behavior for the past 6 months. On some days the patient behaves as usual but on other days, she is irritable and cannot recognize her daughter. This pattern is consistent with fluctuating cognition.
   - She also claims that she sometimes sees two tigers at home which suggests she is experiencing visual hallucinations.
   - Three months ago, she started expressing postural instability, shuffling gait, and the resting tremor. These are signs of Parkinson's disease.
   - Dementia with fluctuating cognition and visual hallucinations along with Parkinsonian features suggests the diagnosis of dementia with Lewy bodies.
   - Dementia with Lewy bodies is commonly accompanied by REM sleep behavior disorder. This is when the patient gains motor control over their body during REM sleep and acts out dreams by moving, talking, or shouting.

3. A 79-year-old man is brought to the physician by his son due to inappropriate behavior for the past 6 months. He makes sexually insulting comments to other family members. He has become irritable and rude. The patient also commonly forgets the names of his family members. MRI of the brain shows bilateral atrophy of the temporal and frontal lobes. He dies 2 years after the initial presentation. What is likely to be found on the autopsy of this patient?
   - **The autopsy of this patient is likely to show Pick bodies in the cerebral neurons.**
   - This patient presents with inappropriate behavior for the past 6 months. He makes sexually insulting comments to other family members. He has become irritable and rude. The patient also commonly forgets the names of his family members. These findings are consistent with the early-onset personality changes along with dementia.
   - His MRI of the brain shows bilateral atrophy of temporal and frontal lobes.
   - All these clues support the diagnosis of frontotemporal dementia, previously known as Pick's disease.
   - Autopsy of the patient with Pick's disease commonly shows round Pick bodies in the cerebral neurons. Pick bodies consist of either hyperphosphorylated tau proteins or ubiquitinated TDP-43.

REVIEW QUESTIONS

4. A 47-year-old man is brought to the physician by his wife due to unusual behavior for the past 2 months. He has become aggressive and rude, and he frequently forgets his children's names. He underwent corneal transplantation 4 months ago. Physical examination shows ataxia and occasional myoclonus. EEG reveals periodic sharp waves. CSF analysis shows increased 14-3-3 protein. What is the most likely pathophysiology of this patient's condition?

    - **The most likely pathophysiology of this patient's condition is conversion of normal prions in α-helix conformation to abnormal prions with β-pleated sheet conformation.**
    - This young patient presents with unusual behavior and memory impairment for the past 2 months. He has become aggressive and rude, and he frequently forgets his children's names.
    - Physical examination shows ataxia and occasional myoclonus.
    - EEG reveals periodic sharp waves.
    - CSF analysis shows increased 14-3-3 protein.
    - All these clues suggest the diagnosis of iatrogenic Creutzfeldt-Jakob disease which is a prion disease.
    - The patient likely developed Creutzfeldt-Jakob disease from his corneal transplantation surgery.
    - Prion diseases are caused by accumulation of abnormal prion proteins in beta-pleated sheet conformation. Abnormal prion proteins then convert the normal prions with alpha-helix conformation into abnormal ones.

5. A 72-year-old man comes to the physician reporting severe forgetfulness for the past 3 months. Once, he forgot to turn off the stove which resulted in a house fire. Sometimes he has trouble remembering his son's name. The patient has been living alone after his wife passed away 6 months ago. He no longer enjoys playing cards with his friends and has trouble falling asleep. The patient feels sad and does not want to get out of bed most days due to him feeling like he moves slower than he used to, to the point that his family has noticed. Which intervention is likely to improve this patient's current condition?

    - **Psychotherapy and antidepressants are likely to improve this patient's current condition.**
    - This patient presents with severe forgetfulness for the past 3 months.
    - He has been living alone since his wife passed away 6 months ago.
    - He no longer enjoys playing cards with his friends. This behavior is consistent with anhedonia.
    - He has trouble falling asleep.
    - The patient also feels sad and does not want to get out of the bed most days due to slowness of movement, which is consistent with psychomotor retardation.
    - Therefore, this patient meets at least 5 criteria of major depressive disorder lasting for at least 2 weeks.
    - Memory impairment in the elderly in the context of depression is called pseudodementia.
    - Pseudodementia along with other signs of depression is likely to improve with psychotherapy and antidepressants.

6. An 88-year-old woman is brought to the physician by her daughter due to gradually worsening memory for the last 3 years. Initially, the daughter thought it was a normal age-related decline but now the patient has severely deteriorated. She cannot recall the names of her family members, and she often gets lost in her neighborhood. Lately, she has become irritable, and she does not talk anymore. Which class of medications is the best initial treatment option for this patient?

    - **The class of medications that is the best initial treatment for this patient is cholinesterase inhibitors.**
    - This elderly patient has had gradually worsening memory impairment for the last 3 years.
    - She cannot recall the names of her family members, and she often gets lost in her neighborhood. Lately, she has become irritable, and she does not talk anymore.
    - Initial symptoms of dementia followed by personality changes and mutism are consistent with the diagnosis of Alzheimer dementia.
    - The best initial treatment options for Alzheimer dementia are cholinesterase inhibitors such as donepezil, rivastigmine, or galantamine.

REVIEW QUESTIONS

7. A 67-year-old man is brought to the physician by his daughter due to gradually worsening memory for the past 3 months. He often forgets the names of his children and grandchildren. The patient also suffers from urinary incontinence. Physical examination shows an abnormal gait with alternating feet sliding on the floor. MRI of the brain shows ventricular enlargement. What is the best next step in management for this patient?

   - **The best next step in management for this patient is a lumbar puncture.**
   - This patient has memory impairment evidenced by forgetting the names of his children and grandchildren. He also suffers from urinary incontinence.
   - The physical exam shows an abnormal gait with alternating feet sliding on the floor. This is consistent with magnetic gait.
   - Brain MRI shows ventricular enlargement.
   - The triad of "wet, wacky, and wobbly" along with ventricular enlargement on MRI of the brain is consistent with the normal pressure hydrocephalus.
   - The best initial management option for patients with the normal pressure hydrocephalus is a lumbar puncture to see if there is improvement in symptoms.
   - If there is an improvement in symptoms, then placement of a ventricular shunt can be considered for long term management.

8. A 65-year-old man is brought to the emergency department by his friend due to severe agitation and aggressiveness for the past 6 months. His past medical history is significant for chronic alcohol use for the past 45 years. The patient tells stories which are inconsistent with what the friend reported. He does not remember his family. The patient's friend says that he used to be a friendly person, but he changed over the course of 2 - 3 years. His vital signs include temperature of 96.8° F (36° C), blood pressure of 135/80 mmHg, heart rate of 81 beats/min, and respiratory rate of 13 breaths/min. Physical examination shows disorientation, abducens nerve palsy, and truncal ataxia. Supplementation of which of the following nutrients could have prevented this patient's current condition?

   A. Cobalamin
   B. Folate
   C. Thiamine
   D. Niacin

- **The correct answer is option C.**
- This patient presents with severe agitation and aggressiveness.
- The patient tells stories which are inconsistent with what the friend reported. This clue suggests the presence of confabulations.
- He does not remember his family, indicative of retrograde amnesia.
- His friend says that he used to be a friendly person, but he changed over the course of 2 - 3 years.
- He has a 45-year-history of alcohol use disorder.
- Confabulations, amnesia, and personality changes in the context of chronic alcohol use are consistent with the diagnosis of Korsakoff syndrome.
- Physical examination shows disorientation, abducens nerve palsy, and truncal ataxia. These signs and symptoms suggest Wernicke's encephalopathy.
- Therefore, this patient has Wernicke-Korsakoff syndrome.
- Although Wernicke's encephalopathy alone is reversible, Korsakoff syndrome is irreversible.
- Wernicke-Korsakoff syndrome is caused by damage to the mammillary bodies and dorsomedial thalamic nucleus due to thiamine deficiency. Therefore, thiamine supplementation could have prevented Korsakoff syndrome in this patient.
- Option A is incorrect because deficiency of cobalamin, or vitamin B_{12}, can result in subacute combined degeneration of the spinal cord and dementia-like symptoms. However B_{12} supplementation cannot prevent Wernicke-Korsakoff syndrome.
- Option B is incorrect because deficiency of folate, or vitamin B_9, results in macrocytic megaloblastic anemia. However, B_9 supplementation cannot prevent Wernicke-Korsakoff syndrome.
- Option D is incorrect because deficiency of niacin, or vitamin B_3, results in Pellagra with diarrhea, dermatitis, and dementia. However, niacin supplementation can not prevent Wernicke-Korsakoff syndrome.

Neurology | Section 10: Altered Mental Status

I. Coma: Definition
   A. A type of altered mental status
   B. Completely unresponsive to stimuli
   C. Impairment of arousal system

Condition	Self-Awareness	Sleep-Wake Cycle	Respiratory Function	Brainstem Reflexes
Brain death	Absent	Absent	Absent	No response
Coma	Absent	Absent	Variably depressed	Intact
Vegetative state	Absent	Intact	Normal	No purposeful response

TABLE 13.1.3 - Brain Death, Coma, and Vegetative State

II. Coma: Etiology
   A. Structural brain lesions (e.g. hematoma, tumors)
   B. Diffuse ischemic encephalopathy, axonal injury
   C. Metabolic disorders (e.g. hyperglycemia, thiamine deficiency)
   D. Infections (e.g. viral encephalitis, bacterial meningitis)
   E. Medications (e.g. benzodiazepines, opiates)

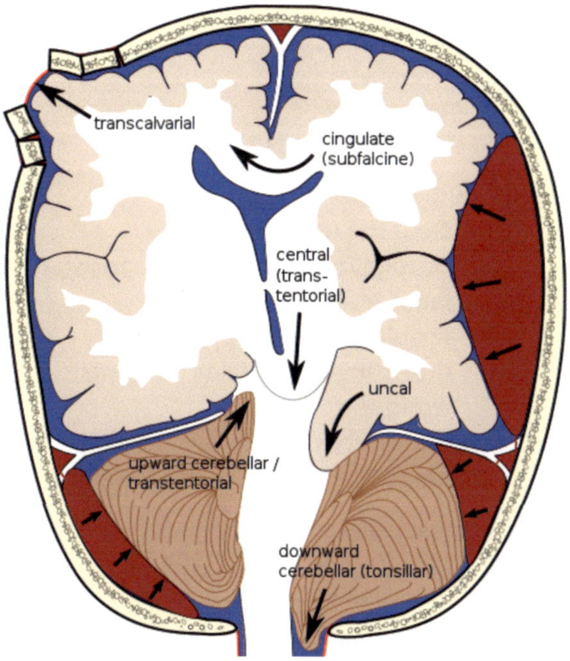

FIGURE 13.1.45 - Types of Brain Herniation

III. Coma: Diagnosis
   A. Assess vital signs
   B. Assess for underlying trauma
   C. Assess consciousness level using the glasgow coma scale
   D. CBC, electrolytes, BUN, creatinine, ABG
   E. ECG
   F. Toxicologic analysis
   G. Imaging (e.g. CT)
   H. Lumbar puncture

	Eye	Verbal	Motor
1	Does not open	No sounds	No movements
2	Open eyes to pain	Makes sounds	Extension to painful stimuli
3	Open eyes to voice	Speaks words	Abnormal flexion to painful stimuli
4	Open eyes spontaneously	Confused/ disoriented	Withdrawal from painful stimuli
5	NA	Oriented	Localizes the painful stimuli
6	NA	NA	Obeys commands

TABLE 13.1.4 - Glasgow Coma Scale

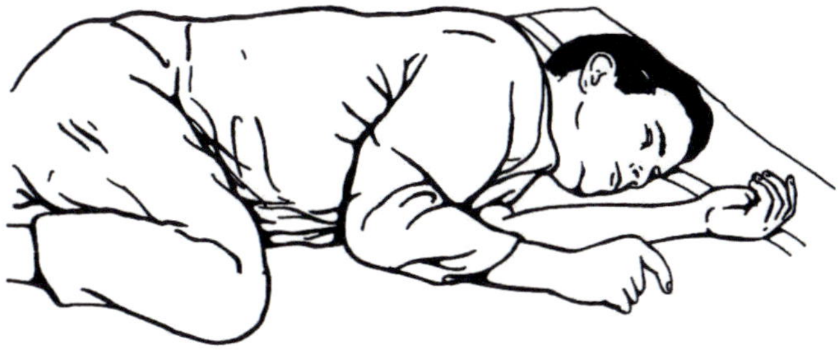

FIGURE 14.1.46 - Lateral Positioning

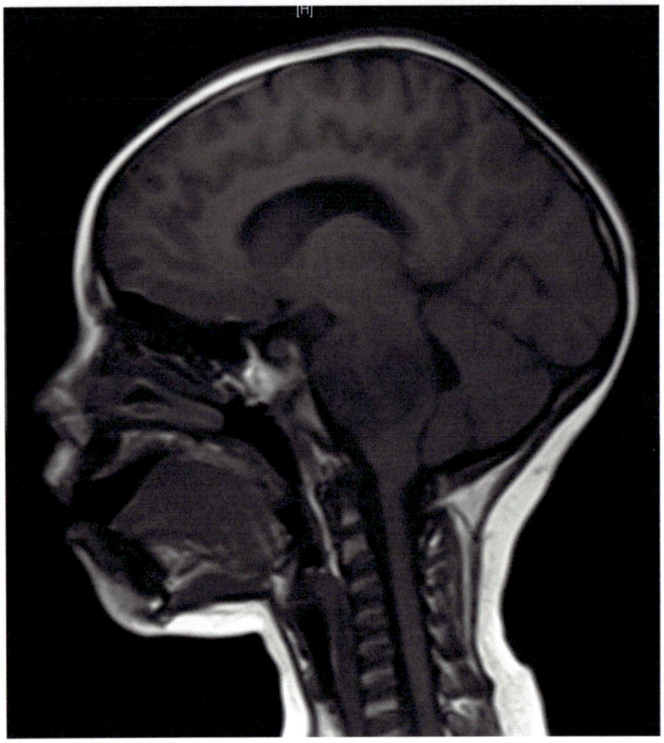

Tdvorak, CC BY-SA 3.0 <https://creativecommons.org/licenses/by-sa/3.0>, via Wikimedia Commons

FIGURE 13.1.47 - MRI of the Head: Glioma

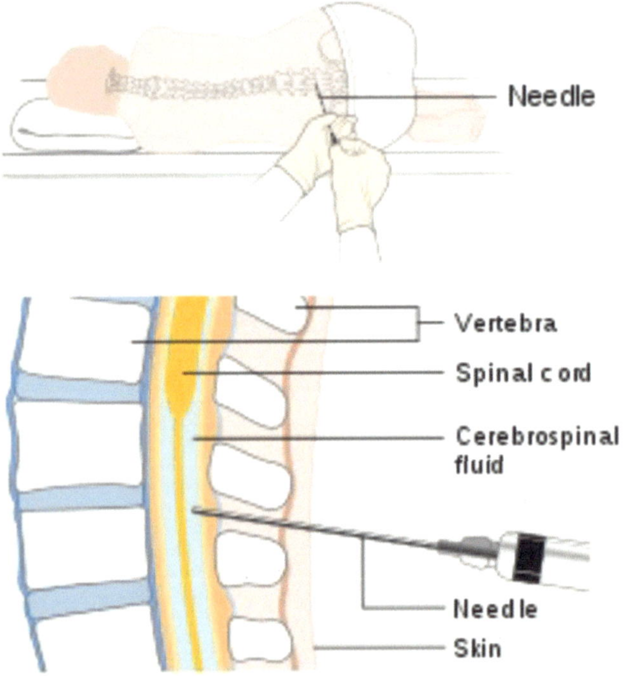

Cancer Research UK, CC BY-SA 4.0 <https://creativecommons.org/licenses/by-sa/4.0>, via Wikimedia Commons

FIGURE 13.1.48 - Lumbar Puncture

IV. Coma: Management
   A. Airway, breathing, circulation (ABC)
   B. Naloxone (opioid overdose), thiamine and dextrose (alcoholic)
   C. Constant monitoring

V. Delirium: General Characteristics
   A. Acute cognitive dysfunction
   B. Develops over a short period
   C. Usually reversible
   D. Most common in elderly patients

VI. Delirium: Etiology
   A. Infections (e.g. UTIs)
   B. Medications (e.g. narcotics)
   C. Stroke, heart disease, seizures, hepatic and renal disorders
   D. Electrolyte imbalances
   E. Alcoholism
   F. Post-operative

VII. Delirium: Clinical Presentation
   A. Rapid deterioration in mental status (vs. dementia)
   B. Fluctuating level of consciousness
   C. Disoriented but alert
   D. Visual hallucinations
   E. Hyperactive or hypoactive
   F. Preexisting cognitive impairment may be present

VIII. Delirium: Diagnosis
   A. History and neurological examination
   B. Work-up
      1. CBC
      2. Electrolytes
      3. Troponins, ECG
      4. Urinalysis

IX. Delirium: Treatment
   1. Treat the underlying cause
   2. Hospitalization, frequent reorientation, familiar faces and objects
   3. Regular sleep-wake cycle
   4. Correcting sensory impairments
   5. Avoid restraints
   6. Antipsychotics (e.g. haloperidol), benzodiazepines (for delirium tremens)

X. Alcohol Withdrawal: Definition
   1. Cessation of alcohol intake after a long period of heavy drinking
   2. Delirium tremens is the most serious form (altered mental status with sympathetic hyperactivity)

XI. Alcohol Withdrawal: Clinical Presentation
   1. Variable onset and duration
   2. Tachycardia, tremors, anxiety, nausea, insomnia
   3. Impaired consciousness
   4. Psychomotor agitation
   5. Auditory and visual hallucinations
   6. Seizures

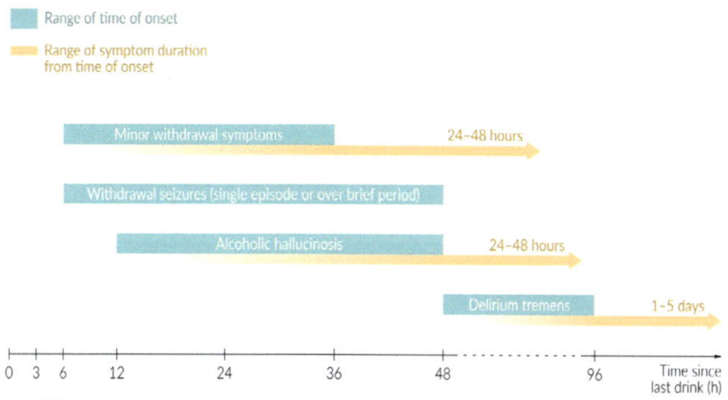

FIGURE 13.1.49 - Features of Alcohol Withdrawal

XII. Alcohol Withdrawal: Diagnosis
   A. DSM-5 criteria of alcohol withdrawal syndrome
   B. Others: CBC, BMP, electrolytes

XIII. Alcohol Withdrawal: Treatment
   A. Benzodiazepines
   B. Supportive therapy (e.g. IV fluids, folate, thiamine, dextrose, multivitamins)
   C. Antipsychotics
      1. Haloperidol
      2. Risperidone

REVIEW QUESTIONS

1. A 70-year-old man is brought by ambulance to the emergency department because of altered mental status for an unknown period of time. His daughter came to visit him this morning and noticed he was confused. Physical examination shows he has slurred speech, ataxia, as well as a nystagmus. The daughter states her father has been a chronic alcoholic for as long as she can remember. What is the most likely diagnosis?
   - **The most likely diagnosis is Wernicke's encephalopathy.**
   - This patient has confusion and ataxic along with a nystagmus.
   - The triad of nystagmus, ataxia, and confusion is a classical presentation of Wernicke's encephalopathy, which results from a thiamine deficiency.
   - The lack of thiamine available to act as a cofactor in glucose metabolism leads to neuronal damage.
   - There is nothing special about alcohol that leads to thiamine deficiency, except that chronic alcoholism is a common cause of malnutrition. This is because patients consume alcohol instead of food.

2. A 30-year-old man is brought to the emergency department by ambulance after being found unresponsive by his partner. Physical examination shows no response to painful stimuli, and he does not open his eyes, he is however making incomprehensible groans. What is the best next step in management?
   - **The best next step in management is to follow the ABCs - A being airway therefore because this patient is unable to protect his airway (indicative because his Glasgow coma score less than 8) he should be intubated.**
   - For the ABCs, the primary decision point is whether or not this person needs to be intubated.
   - A guideline is using the glasgow coma scale, and the general principle is that a score of less than 8 requires intubation.
   - This patient does not open eyes to painful stimuli, which means he gets 1 point; incomprehensible groans are 2; and not withdrawing from the stimulus is 1.
   - This patient has a GCS of 4, which means this patient needs intubation for airway protection.

REVIEW QUESTIONS

3. An 85-year-old woman is brought to the emergency department by her daughter who states that her mother was acting very odd this afternoon. The daughter states that her mother was completely normal yesterday. The patient is unable to state the year, where she is, or why she is here, but does say that she is feeling a little tired. What initial work up should the physician order?

- **The physician should order CBC, electrolytes, troponins, ECG, urinalysis, and medications review.**
- This elderly patient presents with a change in mental status, which can be due to various causes.
- Workup of acute altered mental status should begin with CBC, electrolytes, troponins, ECG, urinalysis, and medications review.
- Further workup is directed at the underlying causes. For example, chest X-ray for suspected pneumonia or head CT for a suspected stroke.

4. A 63-year-old man is admitted to the hospital for an elective ankle replacement. He has a history of degenerative joint disease. He denies alcohol, or drug use. A few hours after an uneventful surgery, the patient becomes agitated. He is confused and inattentive to the hospital staff's questions. He remembers his name, but does not believe that he is in a hospital. What is the best initial treatment option for this patient's underlying diagnosis?

    A. Haloperidol
    B. Allow wife back
    C. Cholinesterase inhibitors
    D. No treatment

- **The correct answer is option B.**
- This patient experiences agitation and confusion right after surgery.
- This is a case of acute-onset altered mental status. Postoperative delirium is the most likely diagnosis.
- First-line treatment for delirium is treating the underlying cause.
- For this patient, where the cause is likely coming out of anesthesia, the underlying cause cannot be changed.
- However, frequently reorienting the patient and seeing familiar faces will usually help.
- Option A is incorrect because haloperidol may be used to treat a brief psychotic episode. For delirium, use of medications or restraints are last-line treatments.
- Option C is incorrect because cholinesterase inhibitors can be used in the treatment of dementia which is a chronic disease with an insidious onset and a progressive course.
- Option D is incorrect because this patient is experiencing distress and the hospital staff should do what they can to alleviate it.

Neurology | Section 11: Demyelinating Disease

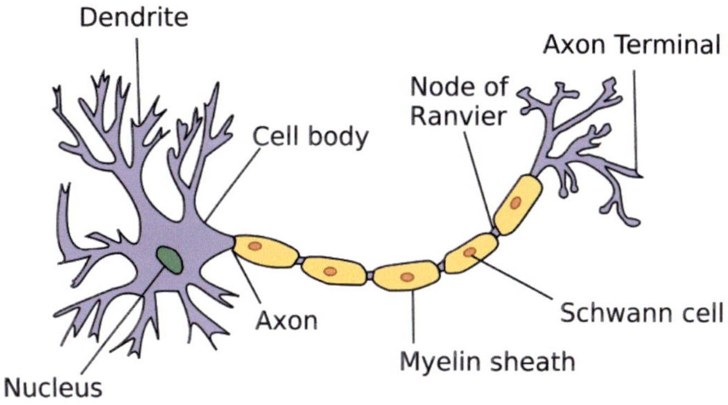

FIGURE 13.1.50 - Neuron Structure

I. Multiple Sclerosis: Definition
   A. Demyelinating disorder of the central nervous system
   B. Primarily affects the white matter of the brain and the spinal cord

II. Multiple Sclerosis: Pathophysiology
   A. A combination of genetic, environmental, and immunologic factors results in destruction of myelin in the central nervous system
   B. The disorder affects nerves seemingly at random, causing neurological symptoms which cannot be explained by a single lesion

III. Multiple Sclerosis: Risk Factors
   A. Young, caucasian woman
   B. Living far away from the equator
   C. Vitamin D deficiency
   D. HLA-DRB1
   E. Smoking
   F. EBV

IV. Multiple Sclerosis: Clinical Presentation
   A. Recurrent neurological symptoms "separated by space and time"
   B. Lhermitte sign
   C. Uhthoff phenomenon
   D. Bilateral trigeminal neuralgia
   E. Transverse myelitis
   F. Optic neuritis
   G. Internuclear ophthalmoplegia

V. Optic Neuritis
   A. Painful, unilateral vision loss due to immune-mediated demyelination of the optic nerve
   B. "Washed-out color vision" or "red color desaturation"
   C. Central scotoma
   D. Physical exam reveals relative afferent pupillary defect
   E. Diagnosis with MRI
   F. Treatment with IV steroids

VI. Internuclear Ophthalmoplegia
   A. Lesion in a medial longitudinal fasciculus causes
      i. Diplopia
      ii. Inability to adduct ipsilateral eye
      iii. Nystagmus on abduction of contralateral eye
         a. Cannot adduct left eye = left internuclear ophthalmoplegia
         b. Cannot adduct right eye = right internuclear ophthalmoplegia

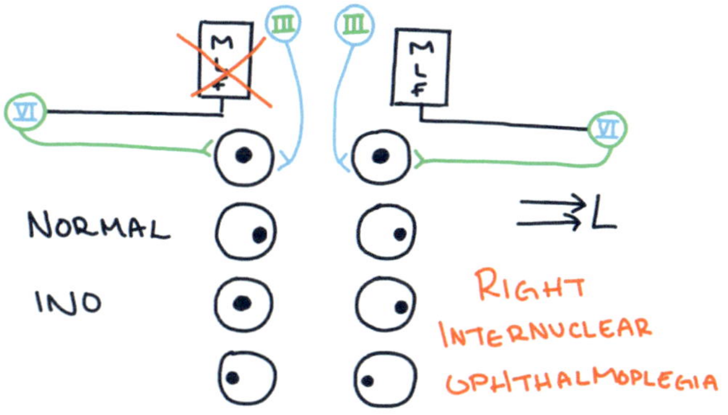

FIGURE 13.1.51 - Right Internuclear Ophthalmoplegia

VII. Multiple Sclerosis: Diagnosis
   A. Clinical diagnosis
   B. MRI: most sensitive test
      1. Periventricular demyelinating plaques
   C. CSF analysis
      1. Oligoclonal bands
   D. Evoked potentials

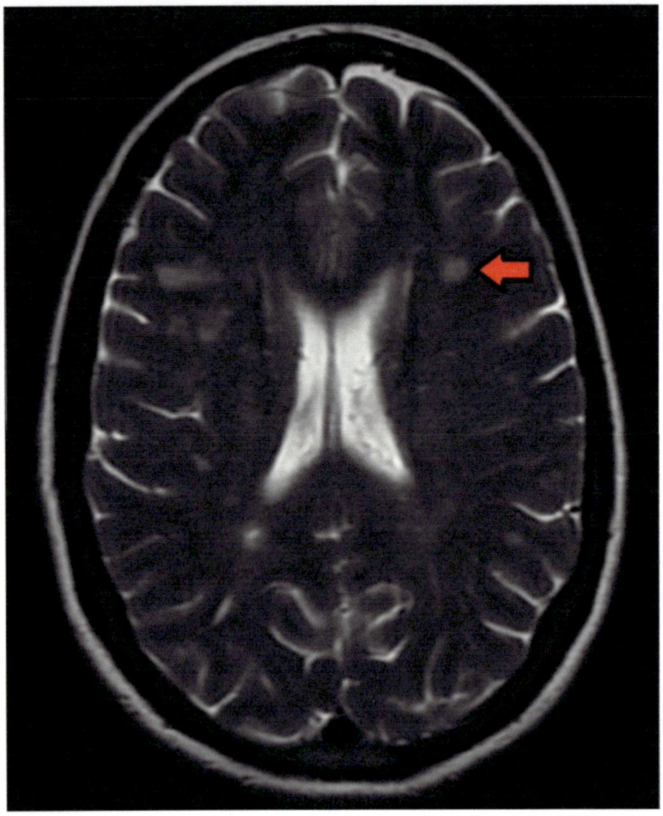

FIGURE 13.1.52 - MRI of the Brain: Multiple Demyelinating Plaques in Multiple Sclerosis

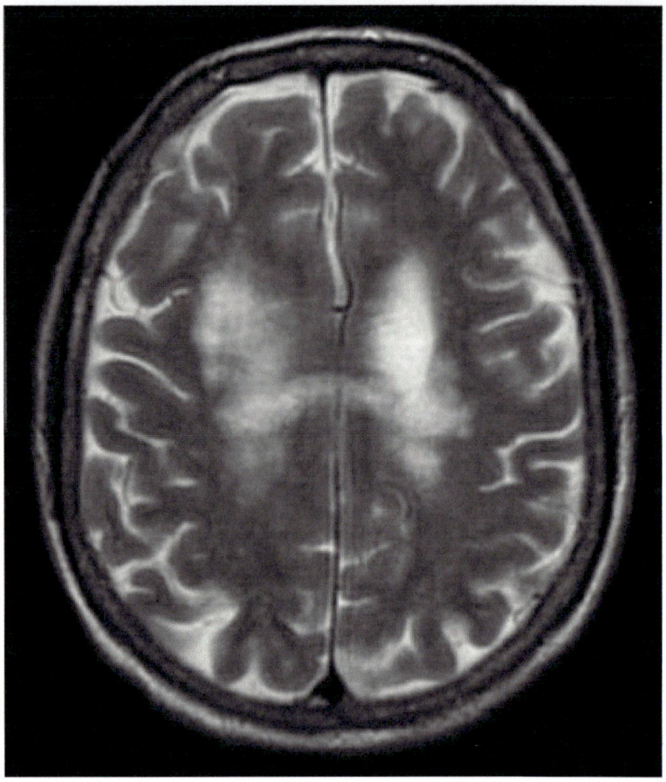

FIGURE 13.1.53 - MRI of the Brain: Demyelination in Progressive Multifocal Leukoencephalopathy

VIII. Multiple Sclerosis: Management
   A. Acute flares: IV steroids, plasma exchange, IVIG
   B. Chronic disease: interferon-beta, natalizumab, and glatiramer
   C. Symptom control
      1. Spasticity treated with baclofen or dantrolene
      2. Trigeminal neuralgia treated with carbamazepine
      3. Depression treated with cognitive behavioral therapy or SSRIs/SNRIs

IX. Acute Disseminated Encephalomyelitis
   A. Similar to multiple sclerosis except
      1. Causes encephalopathy
      2. Does not cause chronic disease
   B. Demyelinating plaques in the thalamus are suggestive of ADEM
   C. Typically preceded by infection or immunization
   D. Treatment is with IV steroids

X. Progressive Multifocal Leukoencephalopathy
   A. Demyelinating disorder of the brain associated with JC virus
   B. Risk factors: immunosuppression, natalizumab, and rituximab
   C. Clinical presentation: confusion, ataxia, seizures, weakness
   D. Diagnosis: MRI brain, CSF with JC virus
   E. Often fatal
   F. Treat patients with AIDS with antiretroviral therapy

XI. Guillain-Barré Syndrome: Definition
   A. Autoimmune inflammatory demyelinating polyneuropathy that affects the peripheral nervous system
   B. Multiple variants of disease exist
      1. Acute inflammatory demyelinating polyneuropathy
      2. Chronic inflammatory demyelinating polyneuropathy
      3. Miller-Fisher syndrome

XII. Guillain-Barré Syndrome: Pathophysiology
   A. Environmental antigen triggers an immune response against the myelin sheath of peripheral nerves
   B. Destruction of myelin sheath leads to neurologic symptoms

XIII. Guillain-Barré Syndrome: Risk Factors
   A. Infection (e.g. *campylobacter jejuni*, viral infection)
   B. Immunization (e.g. influenza vaccine)

XIV. Guillain-Barré Syndrome: Clinical Presentation
   A. Ascending, symmetric weakness or paralysis
   B. Areflexia
   C. Respiratory arrest
   D. Dysautonomia
   E. Paresthesias

XV. Guillain-Barré Syndrome: Diagnosis
   A. Clinical diagnosis
   B. CSF analysis: albuminocytologic dissociation
   C. Nerve conduction studies: decreased nerve conduction velocity

XVI. Guillain-Barré Syndrome: Management
   A. IVIG and plasmapheresis: first-line
   B. Ventilator support
      1. Monitor negative inspiratory force (NIF) and vital capacity regularly
   C. Physical therapy and rehabilitation
   D. Steroids not helpful
   E. Recovery may take up to a year

XVII. Chronic Inflammatory Demyelinating Polyneuropathy
   A. Guillain-Barré syndrome that lasts > 2 months
   B. Treatment is with IVIG, plasmapheresis, and steroids

XVIII. Miller-Fisher Syndrome
   A. Classic triad: external ophthalmoplegia, ataxia, and areflexia
   B. Anti-GQ1B antibody
   C. Management similar to Guillain-Barré syndrome

REVIEW QUESTIONS ?

1. A 30-year-old woman with a history of multiple sclerosis comes to her primary care physician with concerns of double vision for 1-month. When asked to look to the right, her left eye is not able to move past the midline and there is notable nystagmus visible in the right eye. What is the most likely diagnosis?
   - **The most likely diagnosis is left-sided internuclear ophthalmoplegia.**
   - Caused by damage to the medial longitudinal fasciculus which is the connection between CN VI and CN III.
   - Ultimately damage to the medial longitudinal fasciculus leads to impaired lateral gaze as the adduction of the eye ipsilateral to the lesion is impaired.
   - In this case the patient has a left Internuclear ophthalmoplegia caused by damage to the left medial longitudinal fasciculus.

2. A 35-year-old woman with a history of multiple sclerosis is brought to the emergency department by her husband 30 minutes after a seizure. Her husband states that she did lose consciousness after seizing for 2-3 minutes. She has never had a seizure before. He states she's been experiencing progressive confusion, weakness, and problems with coordination over the past several weeks. She recently started a new medication for multiple sclerosis. He says she's never had neurological symptoms to this extent in the past and was "doing well" prior to starting the new medication. What is the most likely diagnosis?
   - **The most likely diagnosis is progressive multifocal leukoencephalopathy.**
   - This patient with multiple sclerosis is experiencing worsening of neurological symptoms following initiation of a new medication.
   - Since the patient was "doing well" prior to initiation of the medicine, it is unlikely that she had an acute flare of multiple sclerosis or required additional therapy for symptomatic management. Hence, she was most likely initiated on a medicine aimed at controlling the chronic course of her disease.
   - Examples of such medicines are interferon-beta, glatiramer, and natalizumab.
   - Natalizumab has a potential of causing progressive multifocal leukoencephalopathy, which is the likely explanation for her worsening neurological symptoms.

REVIEW QUESTIONS

3. A 25-year-old woman is brought to the emergency department after sudden-onset weakness in her right leg. Patient interview is largely unremarkable aside from she says she went on a camping trip over the weekend with some friends. Physical examination of the right lower extremity shows a 0/5 strength and absent patellar and achilles reflexes. What is the next best step in management?

   - **The next best step is looking for a tick and, if found, carefully removing it with a pair of tweezers.**
   - This patient presents with asymmetric, sudden-onset weakness.
   - She has a history of camping over the weekend.
   - She most likely has tick-borne paralysis. This occurs when a tick attaches to an unlucky camper and causes essentially an asymmetric variant of Guillain-Barré syndrome.
   - Hence, the next best step in this situation would be to look for a tick and, if found, carefully remove it with a pair of tweezers. Once the tick is removed, the symptoms will resolve soon after.

4. A 43-year-old woman comes to the clinic because of weakness and double vision for several weeks. She says her symptoms have gotten progressively worse over this time. She denies having similar symptoms in the past. She says she does not have any chronic medical conditions and that she has been healthy her whole life. She says she always had good primary care follow-up and even received her flu shot about a month ago. She denies pain with eye movements. She does not take any medications. Vital signs are within normal limits. Physical examination shows she is unable to adduct the left eye and unable to abduct the right eye. Sensation to vibration and pinprick is intact throughout. Strength is 5/5 in upper extremities and 2/5 in lower extremities bilaterally. Patellar and achilles reflexes are absent bilaterally. Analysis of the cerebrospinal fluid is most likely to reveal which of the following?

   A. Elevated white blood cell count, normal protein levels
   B. Elevated white blood cell count, elevated protein levels
   C. Normal white blood cell count, normal protein levels
   D. Anti-GQ1B antibody
   E. Oligoclonal bands

   - **The correct answer is option D.**
   - This patient has recent-onset neurological symptoms following a recent immunization.
   - Immunizations, particularly the influenza vaccine, are associated with Guillain-Barré syndrome and its variants.
   - She hasn't experienced neurological symptoms in the past.
   - Physical examination shows ascending symmetric weakness and areflexia.
   - This patient has external ophthalmoplegia in addition to the usual symptoms of Guillain-Barré syndrome, making Miller-Fisher syndrome the most likely diagnosis.
   - Miller-Fisher syndrome typically presents with a triad of external ophthalmoplegia, areflexia, and ataxia, and it is associated with anti-gq1b antibodies, which is why D is the correct answer.
   - Option E is incorrect because oligoclonal bands are found in cerebrospinal fluid of patients with multiple sclerosis.
   - Option C is incorrect because albuminocytologic dissociation is expected on cerebrospinal fluid analysis of patients with most variants of Guillain-Barré syndrome, including Miller-Fisher syndrome.
   - Albuminocytologic dissociation means elevated protein with a normal cell count. Hence, both options A and B are incorrect as they do not correctly describe the changes described by the term albuminocytologic dissociation.

Neurology | Section 12: Neuromuscular Disease

I. Myasthenia Gravis: Definition
  A. Neuromuscular autoimmune disease causing generalized muscle weakness that worsens with use
  B. Females > males
  C. Affects young, middle-aged women and older men

II. Myasthenia Gravis: Pathophysiology
  A. Autoantibodies against postsynaptic acetylcholine (ACh) at the neuromuscular junction → signal blockage, degradation of receptors, or activation of complement → skeletal muscle weakness
  B. Thymus: production of ACh receptors autoantibodies by T-cells

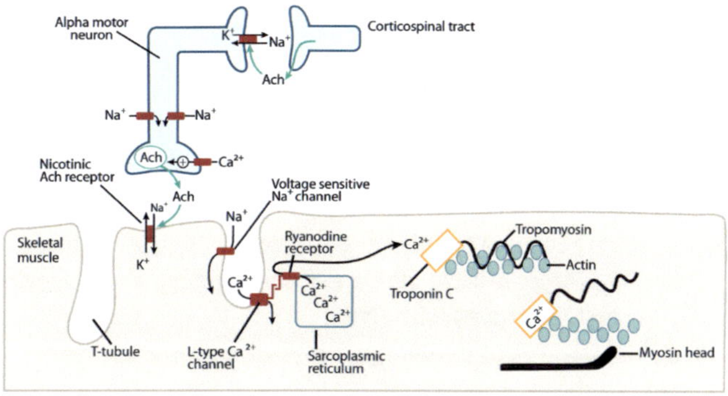

FIGURE 13.1.54 - Neuromuscular Junction

III. Myasthenia Gravis: Risk Factors
  A. Thymoma and thymic hyperplasia
  B. Autoimmune disorders association
    1. Diabetes mellitus (type 1)
    2. Hashimoto's thyroiditis
    3. RA
    4. SLE

IV. Myasthenia Gravis: Clinical Features
  A. Two main clinical forms: ocular and generalized
  B. Ocular: extraocular muscles and eyelid only
  C. Generalized: all skeletal muscles
  D. Muscle weakness and fatigue; worsens with use, improves with rest
  E. Sensation and reflexes are preserved
  F. Eye muscle involvement; usually the first symptoms
    1. Ptosis, diplopia, and blurred vision
  G. Bulbar symptoms
    1. Dysarthria (slurred speech), dysphagia, facial muscles weakness
  H. Respiratory symptoms
    1. Dyspnea, hypoventilation
  I. Limb muscle involvement: proximal and asymmetrical
    1. Difficulty rising from chair, brushing hair
  J. Exacerbating factors
    1. Pregnancy, drugs, infections, surgery
  K. Myasthenic crisis: life-threatening exacerbation
    1. Respiratory muscle weakness and fatigue → respiratory failure

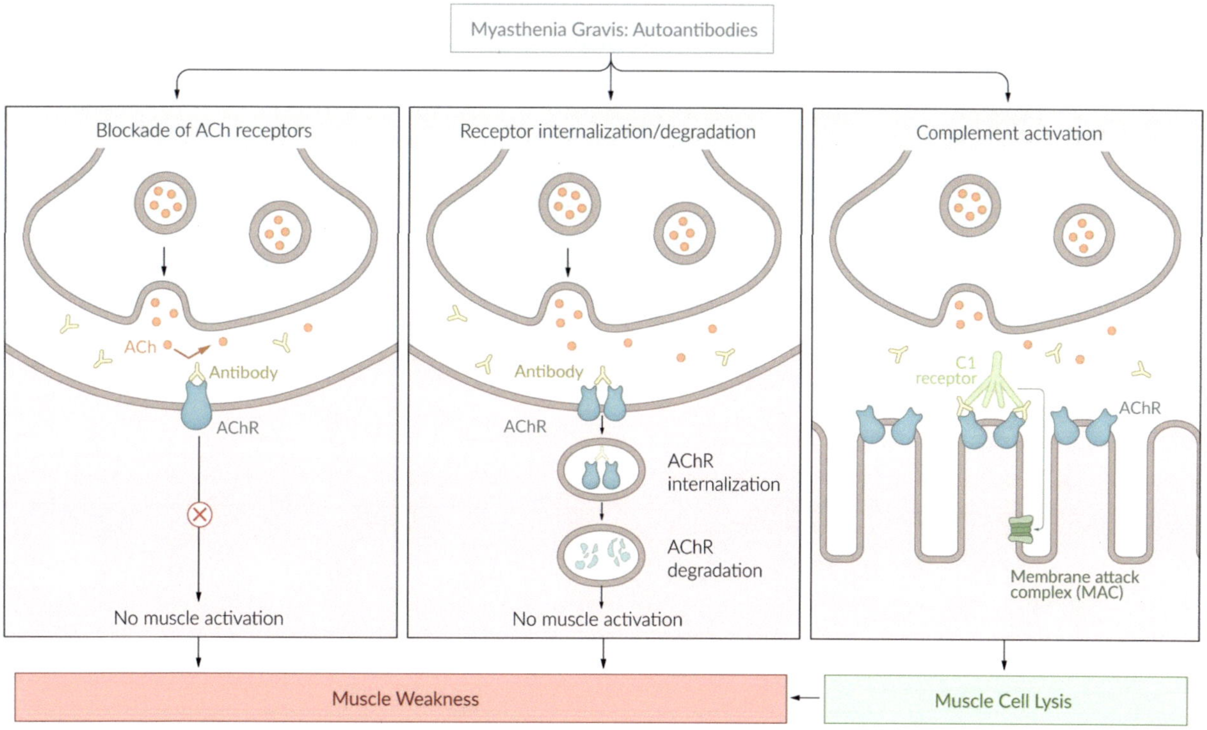

FIGURE 13.1.55 - Pathophysiology of Myasthenia Gravis

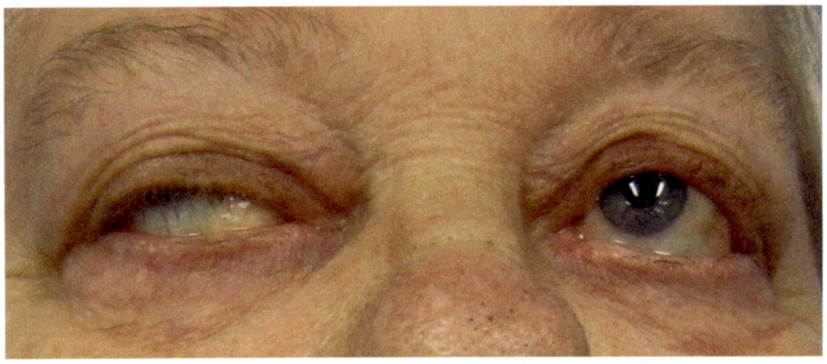

FIGURE 13.5.56 - Ptosis and Strabismus in Myasthenia Gravis

V. Myasthenia Gravis: Diagnosis
   A. Acetylcholine (ACh) receptor antibody test; best initial test
      1. Most specific; could be negative in a small percent of patients
   B. EMG: decremental muscle response upon repetitive stimulation
   C. CT scan: thymoma
   D. Others
      1. Ice test: applying ice over the eyelids improve symptoms
      2. Edrophonium or Tensilon test

VI. Myasthenia Gravis: Management
   A. Myasthenic crisis: endotracheal intubation and mechanical ventilation, plasmapheresis, IVIG; corticosteroids
   B. Cholinesterase inhibitors (e.g. pyridostigmine)
      1. 1st line; symptomatic treatment
   C. Immunomodulators (e.g. glucocorticoids, azathioprine)
   D. IVIG, plasmapheresis
   E. Surgery: thymectomy (if thymoma is present)

VII. Lambert-Eaton Myasthenic Syndrome: Definition
   A. Neuromuscular autoimmune disease causing generalized muscle weakness that improves with use

VIII. Lambert-Eaton Myasthenic Syndrome: Pathophysiology
   A. Autoantibodies against presynaptic voltage-gated Ca^{2+} channels at the neuromuscular junction → ↓ Ca^{2+} influx → disruption of ACh release into the NMJ

IX. Lambert-Eaton Myasthenic Syndrome: Risk Factors
   A. Small cell lung carcinoma-associated paraneoplastic syndrome
   B. Autoimmune disorders association
      1. Diabetes mellitus (type 1)
      2. Hashimoto's thyroiditis
      3. RA
      4. SLE

X. Lambert-Eaton Myasthenic Syndrome: Clinical Features
   A. Proximal muscle weakness and fatigue; worsens with rest, improves with use
   B. Spared extraocular and respiratory muscles; no bulbar symptoms
   C. ↓ or absent reflexes
   D. Autonomic symptoms
      1. Dryness, constipation, orthostatic hypotension

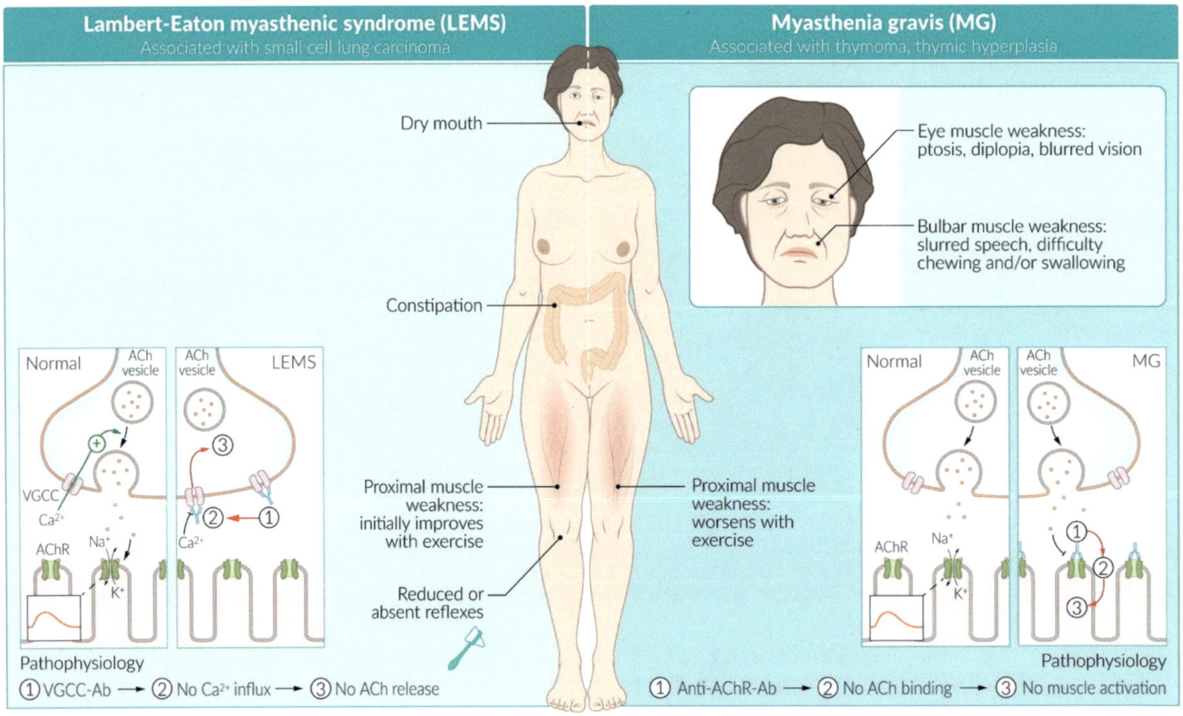

FIGURE 13.5.57 - Myasthenia Gravis vs. Lambert-Eaton Myasthenic Syndrome

XI. Lambert-Eaton Myasthenic Syndrome: Diagnosis
   A. Physical exam
      1. Repetitive muscle use improves the weakness
   B. EMG
      1. Incremental muscle response upon repetitive stimulation
   C. Lab findings
      1. Presynaptic voltage-gated Ca^{2+} channel serum antibodies; confirms diagnosis
   D. CT scan
      1. Small cell lung carcinoma
   E. Others
      1. Edrophonium or Tensilon test

XII. Lambert-Eaton Myasthenic Syndrome: Management
   A. Treat the underlying malignancy, if present
   B. Amifampridine (3,4-diaminopyridine)
      1. 1st line; improves NMJ signal transmission by increasing ACh release from the presynaptic junction
   C. Immunomodulators (e.g. glucocorticoids, azathioprine)
   D. IVIG, plasmapheresis

XIII. Duchenne Muscular Dystrophy: Definition
   A. An X-linked recessive genetic disease that leads to progressive muscle degeneration and weakness
   B. Mostly affects males

XIV. Duchenne Muscular Dystrophy: Pathophysiology
   A. Gene mutation in dystrophin encoding genes → absent dystrophin protein (structural protein) → muscles cell death

XV. Duchenne Muscular Dystrophy: Clinical Features
   A. Progressive muscle weakness and atrophy
      1. Symmetrical
      2. Manifests early in childhood (age 2-3)
      3. Children often need wheelchairs by the age of 12 due to complete loss of ability to walk
      4. Mainly pelvic girdle → progresses to respiratory muscle failure
      5. Gower's sign
   B. Decreased reflexes
   C. Gait disturbances: waddling gait
   D. Pseudohypertrophy of the calf: muscles replaced with fat
   E. Dilated cardiomyopathy: common cause of death
   F. Intellectual disabilities, scoliosis
   G. Late stages: dysphagia, GI disturbances (e.g. intestinal pseudo-obstruction)

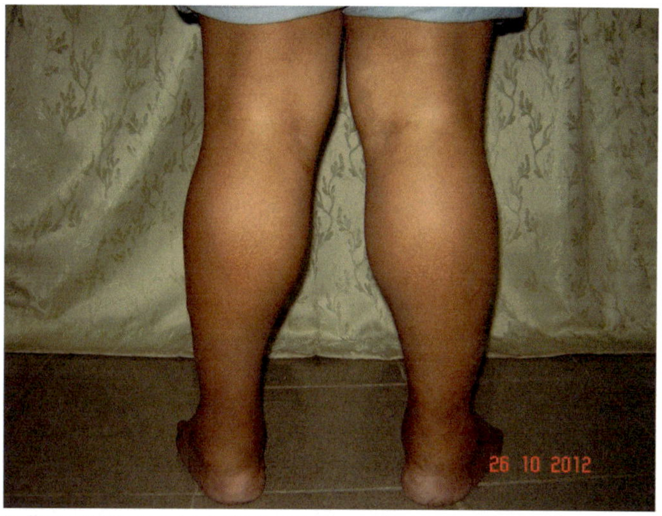

FIGURE 13.5.58 - Pseudohypertrophy of Calf Muscles

	Myasthenia Gravis	Lambert-Eaton Myasthenic Syndrome
Cause	- Thymoma, thymic hyperplasia - Autoimmune diseases	- Paraneoplastic syndrome (small cell lung carcinoma) - Autoimmune diseases
Antibodies	- Against postsynaptic ACh receptors	- Against presynaptic voltage-gated calcium channels
Weakness pattern	- Gets worse with exercise, better with rest	- Gets worse with rest, better with use and exercise
Other key features	- Bulbar symptoms (e.g. dysarthria, facial muscle weakness) - Reflexes preserved - No autonomic symptoms	- No bulbar symptoms - Decreased reflexes - Autonomic symptoms (e.g. dryness, constipation)
EMG	- Decremental response	- Incremental response
Edrophonium or Tensilon test	- Improvement of symptoms	- No response

TABLE 13.1.5 - MG vs LEMS

XVI. Duchenne Muscular Dystrophy: Diagnosis
  A. History and physical exam
  B. Laboratory tests
    1. ↑ serum CK, ↑ serum aldolase
  C. Genetic tests (gold standard): confirms diagnosis; absent dystrophin
  D. EMG
  E. Biopsy: necrotic muscle cells; fat and connective tissue replacing muscle cells

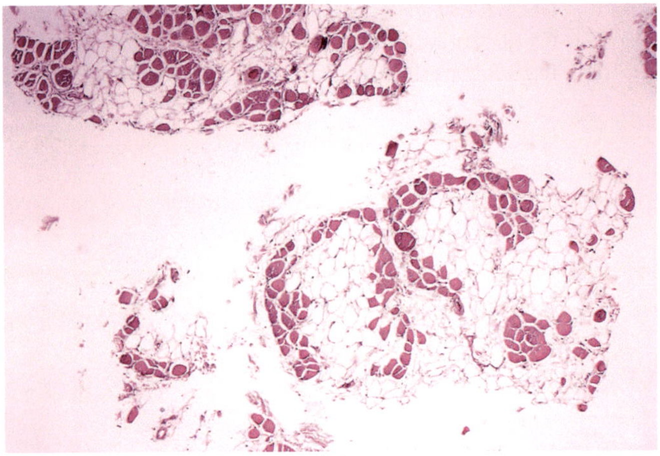

Dr. Edwin P. Ewing, Jr., Public domain, via Wikimedia Commons

FIGURE 13.1.59 - Light Microscopy Replacement of Muscle Tissue by Adipose Tissue in DMD

XVII. Duchenne Muscular Dystrophy: Management
  A. Physical therapy: prevent contractures
  B. Respiratory support
  C. Assisting devices (e.g. wheelchairs)
  D. Surgery: scoliosis correction, contracture release
  E. Glucocorticoids
  F. Prognosis: poor; death usually by 20-30 years of age due to cardiac or respiratory failure

XVIII. Becker Muscular Dystrophy
  A. An X-linked recessive genetic disease that leads to progressive muscle degeneration and weakness; mostly affects males
  B. Pathophysiology similar to DMD, but dystrophin is decreased
  C. Symptoms: similar to DMD, but milder; later onset, slower progression
  D. Diagnosis and management: same as DMD
  E. Prognosis: slightly better than DMD; patient's life expectancy 40-50
  F. Death due to heart failure

	Duchenne Muscular Dystrophy	Becker Muscular Dystrophy
Genetic inheritance	- X-linked recessive	- X-linked recessive
Age of onset	- Earlier (age 2-3)	- Later (age 5-15)
Key features	- Progressive muscle weakness - Scoliosis - Intellectual disabilities	- Milder muscle weakness
Dystrophin	- Absent	- Decreased
Prognosis	- Poor - Wheelchair by adolescence - Death by age 20-30	- Slightly better - Death by age 40-50
Cause of death	- Respiratory failure - Heart failure (dilated cardiomyopathy)	- Heart failure (dilated cardiomyopathy)

TABLE 13.1.6 - Duchenne Muscular Dystrophy vs. Becker Muscular Dystrophy

REVIEW QUESTIONS ?

1. A 37-year-old woman comes to the physician because of progressive muscle weakness and fatigue for the past 3 weeks. She feels like she is more tired by the end of the day, but feels better in the morning. She has smoked a pack of cigarettes daily for the past 20 years. Physical examination shows mild dysarthria and ptosis. Generalized muscle weakness is evident more in the upper limbs. Sensation and deep tendon reflexes are normal. What diagnostic test is most likely to confirm her diagnosis?
   - **AChR antibody test will confirm the diagnosis.**
   - This middle-aged woman presents with generalized, progressive muscle weakness and fatigue.
   - Physical examinations shows ptosis and dysarthria. Sensation and deep tendon reflexes are normal.
   - These findings are consistent with the diagnosis of myasthenia gravis.
   - The test of choice for myasthenia gravis is the acetylcholine receptor antibody test which will confirm the diagnosis.
   - After that, imaging such as a CT scan can be performed to exclude thymoma.

REVIEW QUESTIONS

2. A 5-year-old boy is brought to the physician by his parents because of concerns that he is becoming progressively 'clumsy' for the past 2 months. He started walking later than his older sister around 18 months. He has met all other developmental milestones. Physical examination shows he is pale and anxious. Generalized muscle weakness, as well as enlarged calves bilaterally are noted. When asked to stand from a seated position, he crawls up and puts his hands on his knees for support. This patient is most likely to die from which complication?

    - **This patient is most likely to die from respiratory or heart failure.**
    - This patient has clumsiness and delayed walking.
    - Generalized muscle weakness and enlarged calves are noted. He also presents Gower's sign.
    - These findings are all highly suggestive of duchenne muscular dystrophy.
    - DMD has a poor prognosis and patients usually die due to respiratory or heart failure around 20-30 years of age.

3. A 39-year-old woman is brought to the emergency department via ambulance because of weakness, slurred speech, and difficulty breathing starting 20 minutes ago. She has had an upper respiratory tract infection for the past 2 days and past medical history is notable for early onset rheumatoid arthritis. Her partner notes she has experienced increased muscle weakness for the past 6 months. Physical examination shows difficulty speaking and keeping her eyes open. She appears pale and anxious with blue discoloration of her lips. Vital signs include blood pressure of 116/64 mmHg, pulse of 106 beats/min, temperature of 100.8° F (38.2° C), and respiratory rate of 27 breaths/min with shallow breaths. What is the best next step in the management of this patient?

    A. Pyridostigmine
    B. CT scan
    C. IVIG
    D. Endotracheal intubation
    E. Plasmapheresis

- **The correct answer is option D.**
- This patient has been experiencing increasing muscle weakness for the past 6 months and now she presents with weakness, slurred speech, and difficulty breathing.
- She has had an upper respiratory tract infection for the past 2 days.
- She has a fever, and central cyanosis is noted on physical examination.
- Therefore, this patient is most likely presenting with myasthenic crisis, a life-threatening exacerbation of myasthenia gravis that needs urgent endotracheal intubation.
- Her current symptoms are likely caused by her upper respiratory tract infection which exacerbated the symptoms of undiagnosed myasthenia gravis.
- Hence, she presents with severe respiratory muscle compromise, difficulty breathing, cyanosis (bluish discoloration of her lips), and bulbar symptoms with difficulty speaking and keeping her eyes open.
- Symptoms of myasthenia gravis can be exacerbated by factors such as pregnancy, drugs, infections, and surgery.
- Option A is incorrect because even though pyridostigmine is the mainstay treatment of myasthenia gravis, myasthenic crisis is a life-threatening condition that needs immediate endotracheal intubation.
- Option B is incorrect because even though a CT scan is used to detect thymomas in patients with myasthenia gravis, it wouldn't precede lifesaving measures.
- Options C and E are not the best options because endotracheal intubation is needed first to prevent complete respiratory failure, then plasmapheresis can be done and IVIG can be administered.

Neurology | Section 13: Neurofibromatosis Type I, II and Tuberous Sclerosis

I. Neurofibromatosis Type I: Genetics
   A. Also known as von Recklinghausen disease
   B. Autosomal dominant condition with 100% penetrance
   C. Mutation in *NF1* gene on chromosome 17
      1. *NF1* codes for neurofibromin which normally inhibits RAS protein
      2. Loss-of-function mutation of *NF1* results in disinhibited RAS and unregulated cell proliferation

II. Neurofibromatosis Type I: Clinical Presentation
   A. "CICLOPSS"
      1. Cafe-au-lait spots
      2. Intellectual disability
      3. Cutaneous neurofibromas
      4. Lisch nodules (pigmented iris hamartomas)
      5. Optic glioma and Pheochromocytoma
      6. Seizures (commonly from meningioma) and neurological Signs

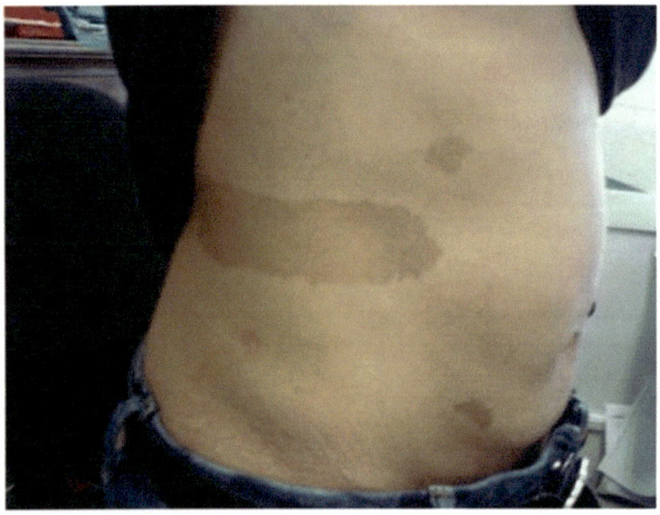

FIGURE 13.1.60 - Cafe-Au-Lait Spots

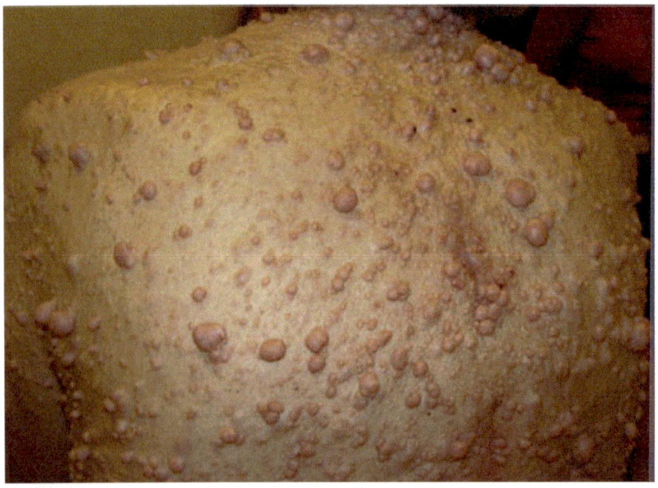

FIGURE 13.1.61 - Cutaneous Neurofibromas

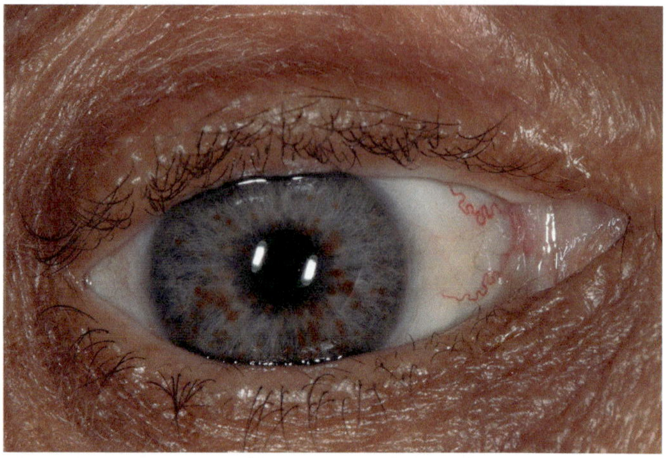

FIGURE 13.1.62 - Lisch Nodules

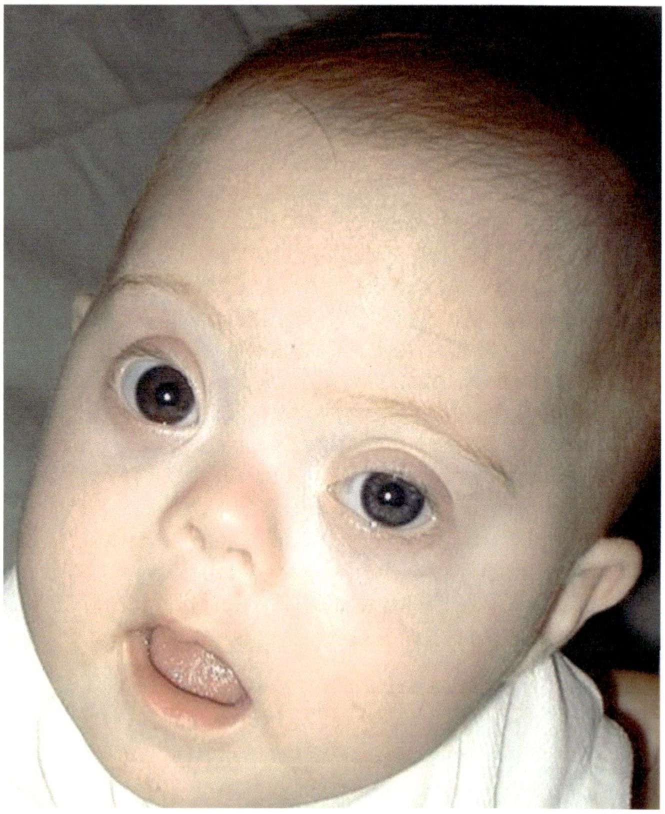

FIGURE 13.1.63 - Brushfield Spots

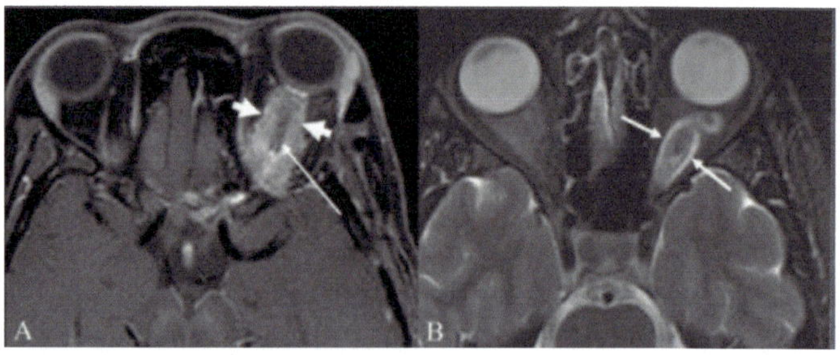

FIGURE 13.1.64 - MRI of the Brain: Optic Glioma

III. Neurofibromatosis Type I: Diagnosis
   A. Based on combination of:
      1. Symptoms and clinical findings
      2. Genetic testing for *NF1* mutation

IV. Neurofibromatosis Type I: Management
   A. Surgical excision of neurofibromas, optic gliomas, meningiomas, and pheochromocytoma
   B. Symptomatic treatment of other clinical features

V. Neurofibromatosis Type II: Genetics
   A. Autosomal dominant condition
   B. Loss-of-function mutation in *NF2* gene on chromosome 22
      1. *NF2* gene codes for merlin (schwannomin) tumor suppressor protein
      2. Loss-of-function mutation inhibits tumor suppression

VI. Neurofibromatosis Type II: Clinical Presentation
   A. Bilateral vestibular schwannomas (acoustic neuromas) with possible sensorineural hearing loss
   B. Juvenile cataracts
   C. Meningioma
   D. Ependymoma

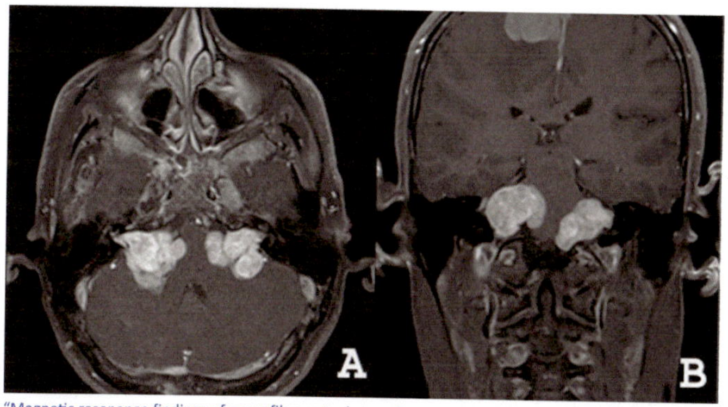

FIGURE 13.1.65 - MRI of the Brain: Bilateral Acoustic Neuromas

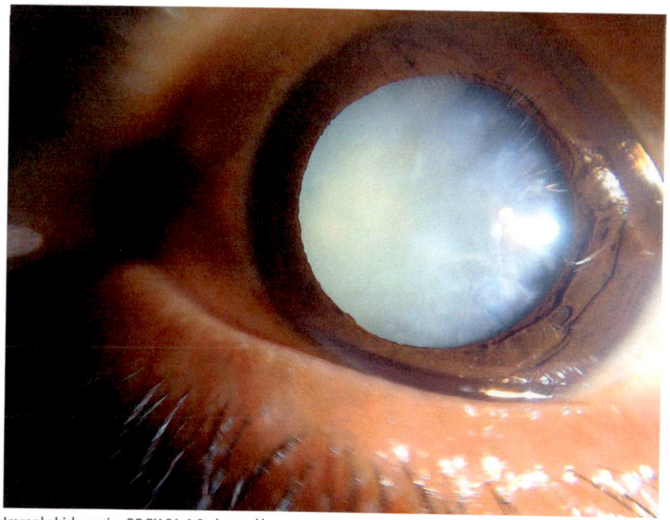

FIGURE 13.1.66 - Cataracts

VII. Neurofibromatosis Type II: Diagnosis
   A. Based on combination of:
      1. Symptoms and clinical findings
      2. Genetic testing for *NF2* mutation

VIII. Neurofibromatosis Type II: Management
   A. Surgery for acoustic neuromas and meningiomas
   B. Radiation for any other tumors
   C. Lens replacement surgery for cataracts

IX. Tuberous Sclerosis: Genetics
   A. Autosomal dominant condition with variable expressivity
   B. De novo mutation is possible
   C. Mutation in tumor suppressor gene *TSC1* on chromosome 9
      1. Codes for hamartin protein
   D. Mutation in tumor suppressor gene *TSC2* on chromosome 16
      1. Codes for tuberin protein

X. Tuberous Sclerosis: Clinical Presentation
   A. "HAMARTOMASS"
      1. CNS and skin **H**amartomas
      2. **A**ngiofibromas (adenoma sebaceum), **M**ental retardation (intellectual disability)
      3. **A**sh-leaf spots, cardiac **R**habdomyoma
      4. **T**uberous sclerosis, autosomal d**O**minant
      5. Renal **A**ngiomyolipomas, **S**eizures, **S**hagreen patches
   B. Increased incidence of:
      1. Subependymal giant cell astrocytoma
      2. Ungual fibromas

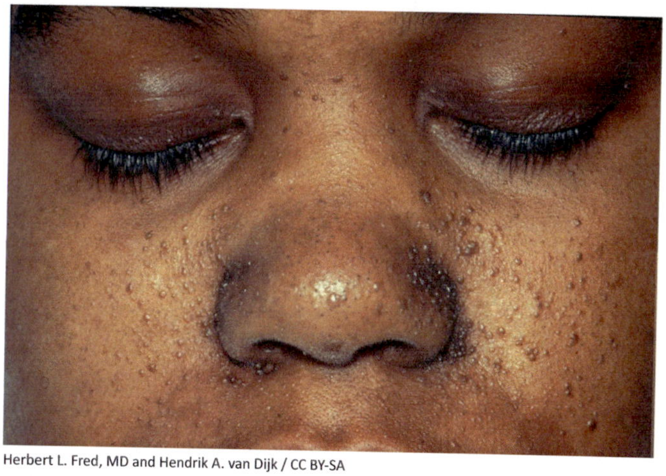

FIGURE 13.1.67- Facial Angiofibromas

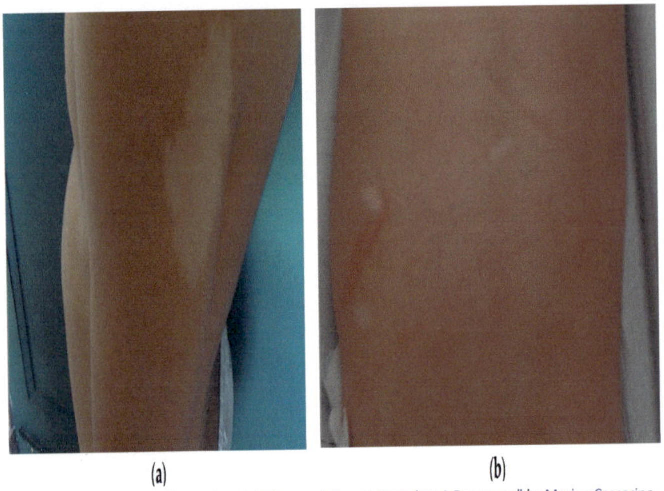

FIGURE 13.1.68 - Ash-Leaf Spot

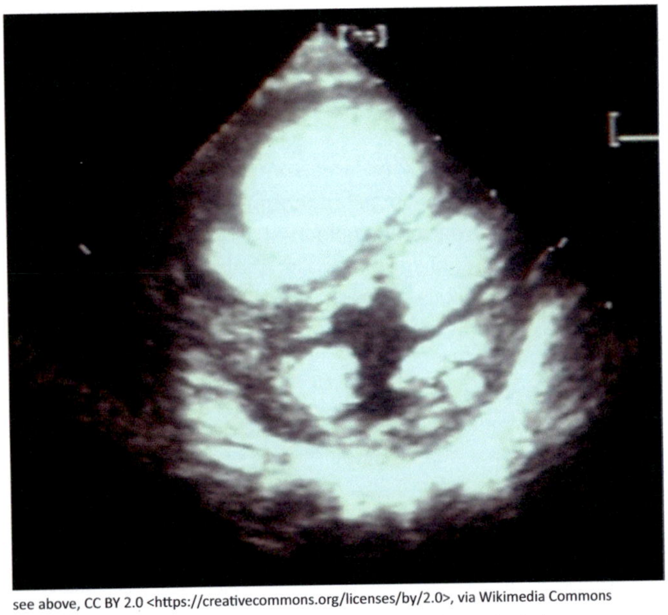

FIGURE 13.1.69 - Echocardiography: Cardiac Rhabdomyoma

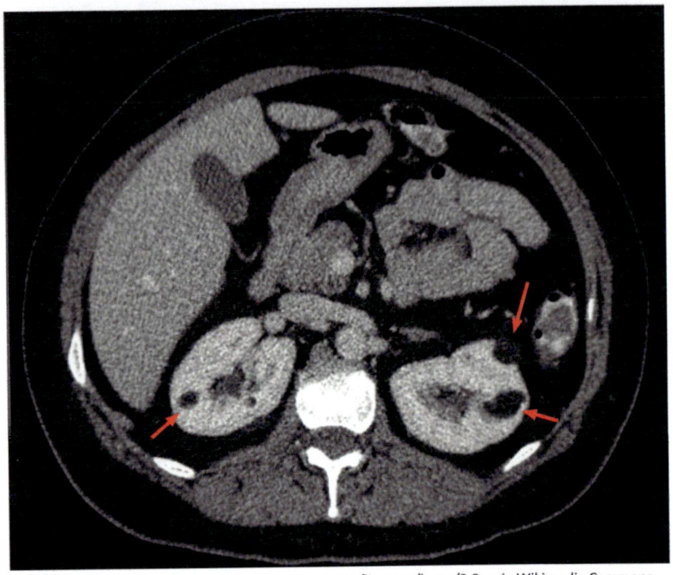

FIGURE 13.1.70 - MRI of the Abdomen: Bilateral Renal Angiomyolipomas

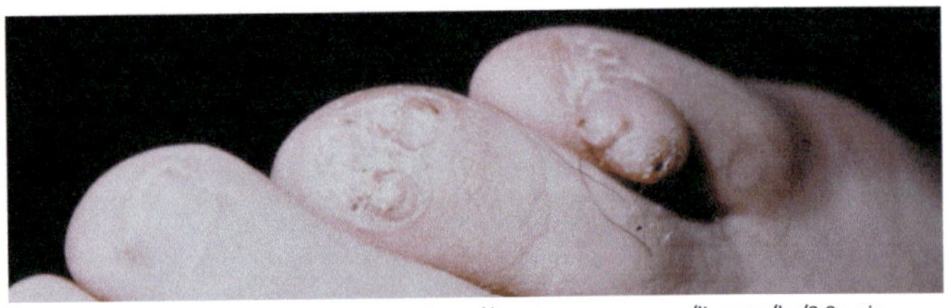

FIGURE 13.1.71 - Ungual Fibroma

XI. Tuberous Sclerosis: Diagnosis
   A. Based on combination of:
      1. Symptoms and clinical findings
      2. Genetic testing for *TSC1*/*TSC2* mutations

XII. Tuberous Sclerosis: Management
   A. Regular skin and eye exams to monitor for tumors
   B. Serial MRI of the brain and kidney
   C. Neuropsychiatric screening
   D. Baseline EEG
   E. Antiepileptics

Condition	Etiology	Key Features
Neurofibromatosis type I (von Recklinghausen disease)	- *NF1* mutation on chromosome 17	- Iris hamartomas (Lisch nodules), neurofibromas, café au lait spots, axillary freckling, bony lesions - Complications: pheochromocytomas and optic nerve gliomas
Neurofibromatosis type II	- *NF2* mutation on chromosome 22	- Bilateral acoustic neuromas (Schwannomas), cafè au lait spots, juvenile cataracts, neurofibromas - Complications: meningiomas, ependymomas, and hearing loss
Tuberous sclerosis	- *TSC1* mutation on chromosome 9 - *TSC2* mutation on chromosome 16	- Ash-leaf spots, shagreen patches, facial angiofibromas, cognitive impairment, epilepsy - Complications: retinal hamartomas, renal angiomyolipomas, and cardiac rhabdomyomas

TABLE 13.1.7 - Neurofibromatosis Type I, Neurofibromatosis Type II, and Tuberous Sclerosis

REVIEW QUESTIONS

1. A 15-year-old boy is brought to the physician by his mother because of three seizures over the last two weeks. His past medical history includes surgery for a left optic glioma. Physical examination shows multiple skin-colored plaques on his back and slightly hyperpigmented patches diffusely on the skin. Fundoscopic exam shows brown nodules bilaterally on the iris. What genetic abnormality is most likely responsible for this patient's condition?

   - **The genetic abnormality responsible for neurofibromatosis type I is a loss-of-function mutation in NF1 gene on chromosome 17.**
   - This patient presents with three seizures over the last two weeks.
   - He has a past medical history of an optic glioma.
   - Multiple skin-colored plaques on his back are most likely neurofibromas, while slightly hyperpigmented patches are cafe-au-lait spots. Brown nodules bilaterally on the iris suggest Lisch nodules.
   - All of these findings are consistent with the diagnosis of neurofibromatosis type I.
   - The genetic abnormality responsible for neurofibromatosis type I is a loss-of-function mutation in NF1 gene on chromosome 17. Therefore, the product of NF1 gene, neurofibromin, can no longer inhibit the RAS protein, which stimulates unregulated cellular proliferation.
   - Loss-of-function mutation in NF1 → ↓neurofibromin → disinhibited RAS protein and unregulated cellular proliferation.

2. A 6-year-old girl is brought to her pediatrician's office by her father because of problems at school for the last month. Her teachers report that she has an extremely hard time following directions. Her past medical history is significant for bilateral lens replacement surgery due to infantile cataracts. Audiometry shows bilateral sensorineural hearing loss. MRI of the brain shows bilateral masses at the cerebellopontine angles. Which central nervous system tumors is this patient at risk for developing?

   - **The two central nervous system tumors that this patient is at risk for developing are meningioma and ependymoma.**
   - This patient is initially evaluated due to inattentiveness at school.
   - She has a past medical history of infantile cataracts.
   - Audiometry shows bilateral sensorineural hearing loss that may be the cause of her behavior at school.
   - MRI of the brain shows bilateral masses at the cerebellopontine angles. This finding is consistent with bilateral vestibular schwannomas.
   - Considering all of these findings, this patient likely has neurofibromatosis type II.

3. A 7-year-old boy is brought to his pediatrician by his parents for a routine well-child visit. He was diagnosed with intellectual disability at the age of 3. He was incidentally found to have bilateral renal masses 2 years ago. The physical exam shows skin-colored nodules around the fingernails, several hypopigmented patches on the trunk, and one large hyperpigmented plaque on his lower back. Echocardiography shows a mass in the left ventricular myocardium obstructing the outflow tract. The cardiac mass is a component of which genetic condition?

   - **The most genetic condition is tuberous sclerosis - cardiac rhabdomyoma.**
   - This patient has an intellectual disability.
   - He was found to have bilateral renal masses two years ago suggesting renal angiomyolipomas.
   - Skin-colored nodules around the fingernails are consistent with ungual fibromas. Hypopigmented patches indicate ash-leaf spots, and one large hyperpigmented plaque on his lower back suggests a Shagreen patch.
   - All of these findings indicate tuberous sclerosis.
   - Echocardiography shows a mass in the left ventricular myocardium obstructing the outflow tract. A myocardial mass in a patient with tuberous sclerosis is most likely a cardiac rhabdomyoma.

Neurology | Section 14: Neurocutaneous Syndromes: Sturge-Weber and von-Hippel-Lindau Syndromes

I. Sturge-Weber Syndrome: Genetics
   A. Congenital non-hereditary condition
   B. Also known as encephalo trigeminal angiomatosis
   C. Affects neural crest cell derivatives
   D. Somatic mosaicism of activating mutation in one copy of *GNAQ* gene
      1. *GNAQ* gene codes for α-subunit of G_q-protein

II. Sturge-Weber Syndrome: Clinical Presentation
   A. Port-wine stain ("nevus flammeus"): capillary malformation in CN V_1/V_2 distribution
   B. Ipsilateral leptomeningeal angioma with "tram-track" calcifications of the gyri
   C. Seizures and intellectual disability
   D. Episcleral hemangioma → ↑ Intraocular pressure → early-onset glaucoma

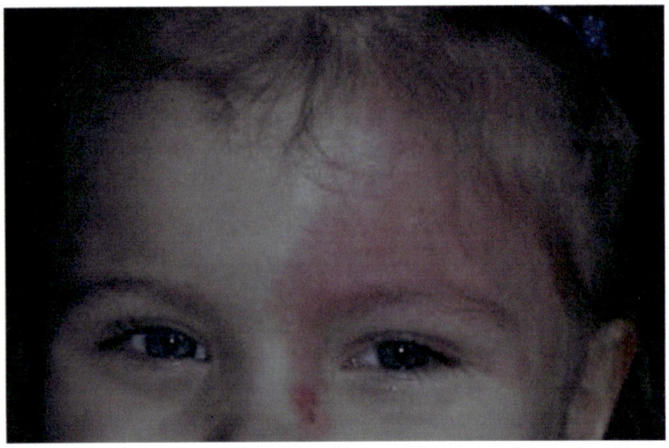

FIGURE 13.1.72 - Port-Wine Stain

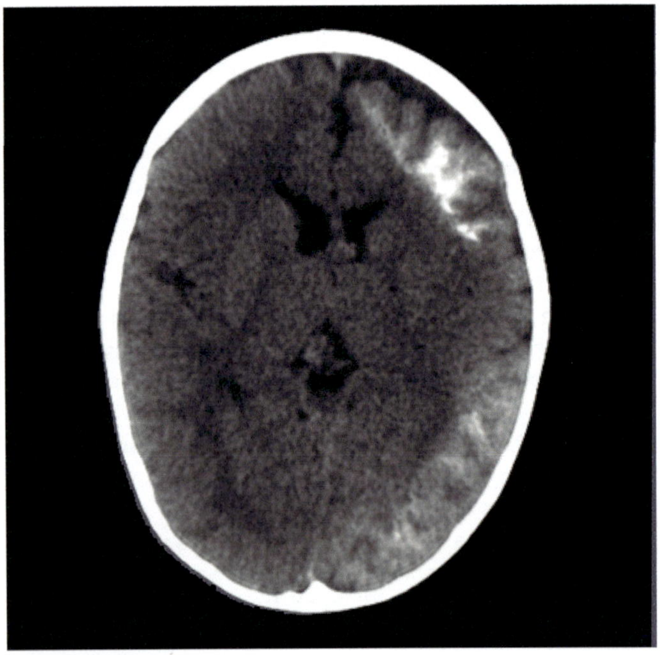

FIGURE 13.1.73 - CT Scan of Head: Leptomeningeal Angiomas with Calcifications

III. Sturge-Weber Syndrome: Diagnosis
   A. Based on combination of
      1. Symptoms and clinical findings
      2. Genetic testing for *GNAQ* mutations (not routinely performed)

IV. Sturge-Weber Syndrome: Management
   A. Antiepileptics for seizures
   B. Pulsed laser therapy for the port-wine stain
   C. Supportive

V. Von-Hippel-Lindau Syndrome: Genetics
   A. Autosomal dominant condition
   B. Deletion of *VHL* gene on chromosome *3p*
      1. *VHL* gene codes for *VHL* protein that ubiquitinates and inactivates hypoxia-inducible factor 1a (transcription factor stimulating vascularization in hypoxic tissues)
      2. *VHL* gene deletion → disinhibited hypoxia-inducible factor 1a → vascular tumors in multiple organ systems

VI. Von-Hippel-Lindau Syndrome: Clinical Presentation
   A. "HARP"
      1. **H**emangioblastoma in retina, brainstem, cerebellum, spinal cord
      2. **A**ngiomatosis
      3. Bilateral **R**enal cell carcinoma
      4. **P**heochromocytomas

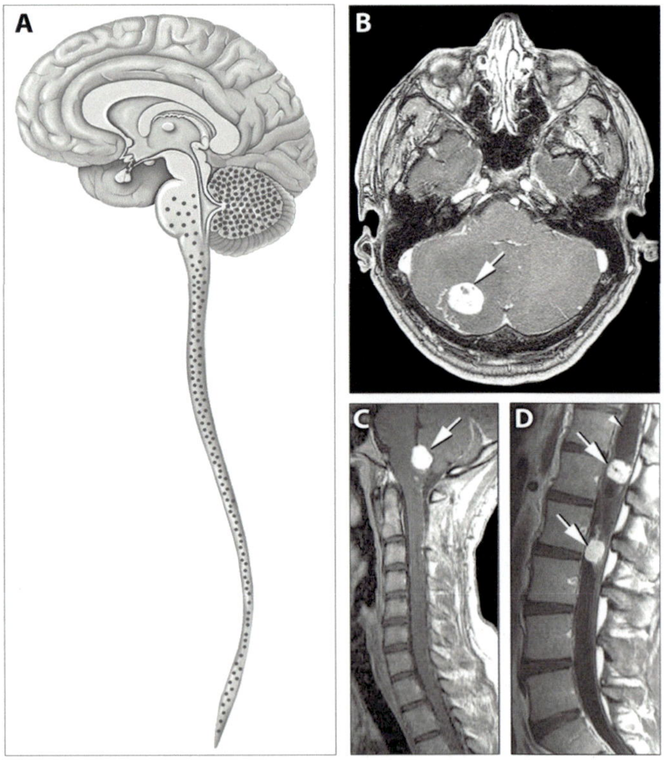

FIGURE 13.1.74 - MRI of the Brain and Spinal Cord: Hemangioblastomas

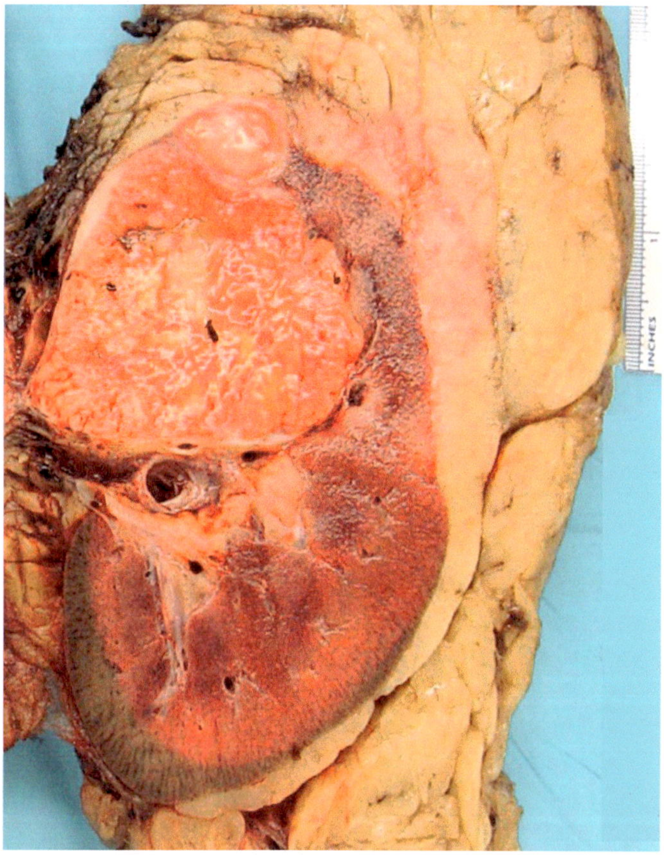

FIGURE 13.1.75 - Renal Cell Carcinoma

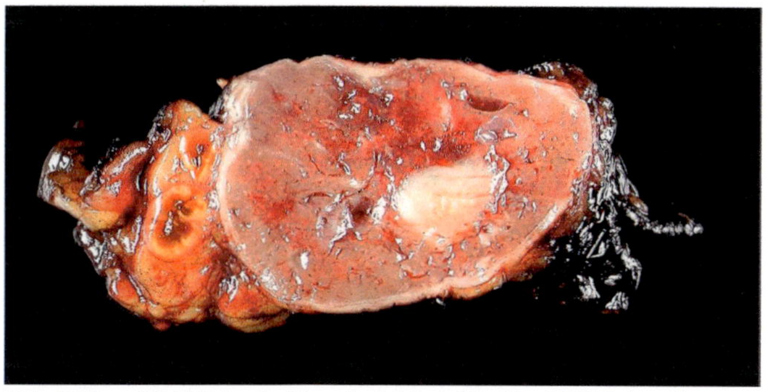

FIGURE 13.1.76 - Pheochromocytoma

VII. Von-Hippel-Lindau Syndrome: Diagnosis
   A. Based on combination of
      1. Symptoms and clinical findings
      2. Genetic testing for *VHL* gene deletion

VIII. Von-Hippel-Lindau Syndrome: Management
   A. Screening for associated tumors (e.g. abdominal ultrasound or CT scan, fundoscopy)
   B. Surgical resection of tumors

Condition	Etiology	Key Features
Sturge-Weber disease	- Sporadic *GNAQ* gene mutation	- Port wine stain, epilepsy, intellectual disability - Complications: capillary angiomatosis of the pia mater
von-Hippel-Lindau disease	- *VHL* gene deletion on chromosome 3p	- Cavernous hemangiomas of the brain or brainstem, renal angiomas, and cysts in multiple organs - Complications: renal cell carcinoma and pheochromocytoma

TABLE 13.1.8 - Sturge-Weber Syndrome and Von-Hippel-Lindau Disease

REVIEW QUESTIONS

1. A 5-year-old girl is brought to the physician by her mother due to worsening left eye pain that started 4 weeks ago. She has a past medical history of intellectual disability and tonic-clonic seizures treated with valproic acid. Physical examination shows a large erythematous patch on the left side of her face involving the forehead, periorbital skin, and the cheek. An MRI of the brain shows a left-sided vascular malformation in the pia mater with calcifications of the gyri. Ophthalmological exam of the left eye shows an intraocular pressure of 40 mmHg (10-21 mmHg). What is the most likely cause of the ophthalmologic exam finding in this patient?

- **The most likely cause is episcleral hemangioma compressing the eyeball.**
- This patient presents with left eye pain.
- Her past medical history includes intellectual disability and tonic-clonic seizures.
- A large erythematous mass involving the forehead, periorbital skin, and cheek is consistent with a port-wine stain, or "nevus flammeus."
- A vascular malformation in the pia mater with calcifications of the gyri suggests leptomeningeal angioma with "tram-track" calcifications.
- All of these findings are consistent with the diagnosis of Sturge-Weber syndrome.
- This patient has an increased intraocular pressure in the left eye. Increased intraocular pressure and resultant glaucoma in patients with Sturge-Weber syndrome are due to an episcleral hemangioma compressing the eyeball.

2. A 14-year-old boy is brought to the primary care physician for a routine examination. He has no specific complaint. His past medical history includes unilateral nephrectomy due to renal cell carcinoma and unilateral adrenalectomy for pheochromocytoma. Two years ago, he was found to have a mass next to the spinal cord after complaining of intractable back pain. Biopsy of the mass showed blood vessels with hyperchromatic nuclei in the cells. Vital signs include temperature of 96.8° F (36° C), blood pressure of 110/80 mmHg, heart rate of 92 beats/min, and respirations of 15 breaths/min. Which of the following is recommended for this patient on a regular basis?

   A. Fundoscopic exam
   B. Complete blood count
   C. TSH levels
   D. Basic metabolic panel

- **The correct answer is option A.**
- This patient has a past medical history of renal cell carcinoma and pheochromocytoma.
- Biopsy of a mass found next to the spinal cord showed vessels with hyperchromatic nuclei in the cells. This is a classic description for hemangioblastoma.
- This patient has a history of renal cell carcinoma, pheochromocytoma, and hemangioblastoma.
- Presence of these tumors at such a young age already increases the suspicion for a genetic syndrome.
- Therefore, the most likely diagnosis is von-Hippel-Lindau syndrome.
- Patients with von-Hippel-Lindau syndrome commonly develop retinal hemangioblastoma. This is why these patients need to undergo regular fundoscopy to check for retinal hemangioblastoma.
- Option B, option C, and option D are all incorrect because none of these tests screen for complications of von-Hippel-Lindau syndrome, and, therefore, are not indicated in these patients on a regular basis.

Neurology | Section 15: Anterior Cord Syndrome, Central Cord Syndrome & Brown-Sequard Syndrome

I. Anterior Cord Syndrome: Definition
   A. Damage of the tracts in the two anterior thirds of the spinal cord
      1. Corticospinal tracts, spinothalamic tracts, descending autonomic tracts

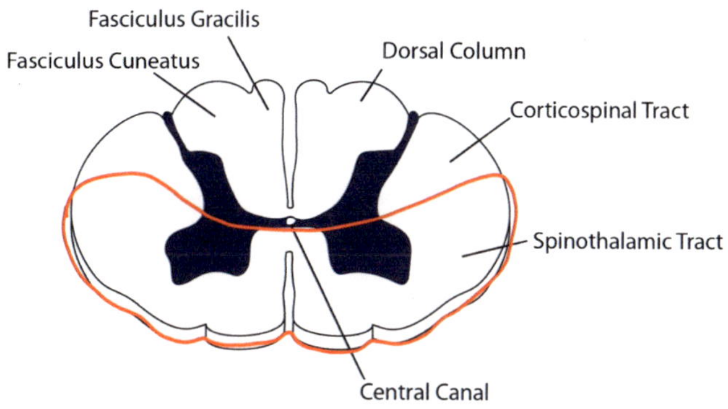

FIGURE 13.1.77 - Cross-Section of the Spinal Cord: Area Affected in Anterior Cord Syndrome

II. Anterior Cord Syndrome: Etiology
   A. Anterior spinal artery injury
      1. Infarction
      2. Intervertebral disc herniation
      3. Vertebral burst fracture
   B. Radiation myelopathy

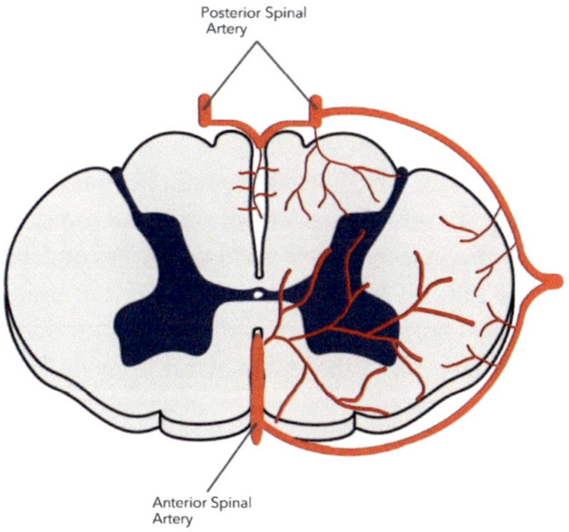

FIGURE 13.1.78 - Anterior Spinal Artery

III. Anterior Cord Syndrome: Clinical Features
   A. Damage of lateral corticospinal tracts
      1. Bilateral hemiparesis at and below lesion level
   B. Damage of lateral spinothalamic tracts
      1. Bilateral loss of pain and temperature sensation below the lesion level
   C. Damage of autonomic tracts (descending to the sacral cord)
      1. Urinary incontinence
   D. Dorsal tracts are intact
      1. Intact bilateral proprioception and vibratory sensation

IV. Anterior Cord Syndrome: Diagnosis and Management
   A. Diagnosis
      1. MRI
   B. Management
      1. Treat underlying cause if applicable
      2. Surgical decompression

V. Central Cord Syndrome: Etiology
   A. The most common among incomplete cord syndromes
   B. Causes
      1. Syringomyelia
      2. Intramedullary tumor
      3. Hyperextension injury in patients with cervical spondylosis

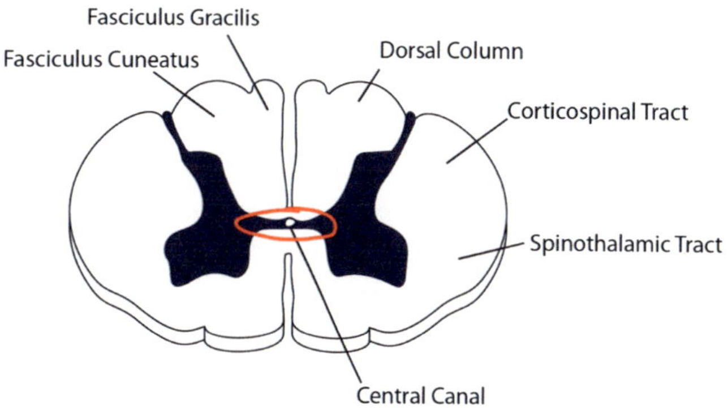

FIGURE 13.1.79 - Cross-Section of the Spinal Cord: Area Affected in Central Cord Syndrome

VI. Central Cord Syndrome: Clinical Features
   A. Damage of spinothalamic fibers in anterior white commissure
      1. Bilateral loss of pain and temperature sensation at lesion level
      2. Normal pain and temperature sensation above and below the injury level (suspended sensory level)
   B. Compressing anterior horn neurons
      1. LMN lesion: flaccid weakness, diminished DTRs at lesion level

VII. Central Cord Syndrome: Diagnosis and Management
   A. Diagnosis
      1. MRI (imaging test of choice)
   B. Management
      1. Treat underlying cause if applicable
      2. Physical and occupational therapy
      3. Surgical intervention

VIII. Brown-Sequard Syndrome: Definition and Etiology
   A. Hemisection of the spinal cord
   B. Etiology
      1. Trauma (penetrating trauma is most common)
      2. Mass lesions (e.g. tumor, hematoma)

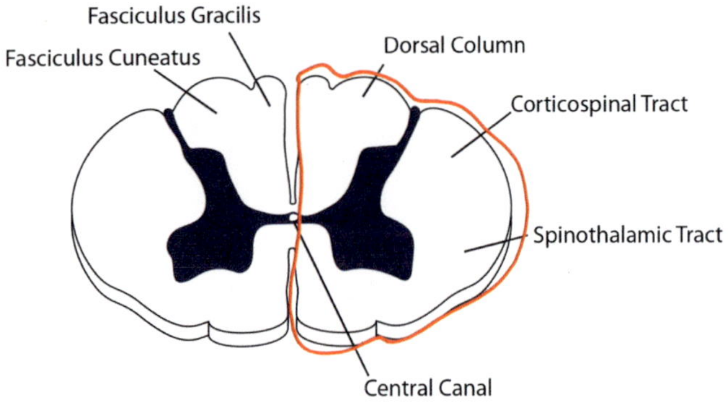

FIGURE 13.1.80 - Cross-Section of the Spinal Cord: Area Affected in Brown-Sequard Syndrome

IX. Brown-Sequard Syndrome: Clinical Features
   A. Damage of lateral corticospinal tracts
      1. Ipsilateral hemiparesis at and below the lesion level
   B. Damage of dorsal columns
      1. Ipsilateral loss of proprioception and vibration sensation at and below the lesion level
   C. Damage of lateral spinothalamic tracts
      1. Contralateral loss of pain and temperature sensation starting 1-2 levels below the lesion
   D. Damage of cervical sympathetic pathways
      1. Ipsilateral horner syndrome
   E. On neurologic examination: sensory level is present

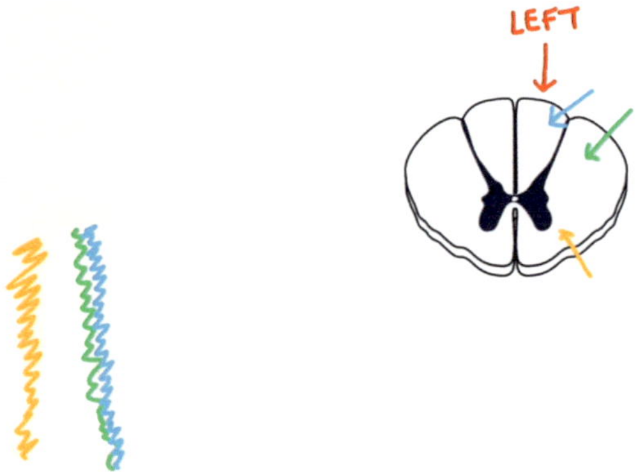

FIGURE 13.1.81 - Brown-Sequard Syndrome

X. Brown-Sequard Syndrome: Diagnosis and Management
   A. Diagnosis
      1. MRI (the imaging test of choice)
   B. Management
      1. Early administration of steroids
      2. Treat underlying cause if applicable
      3. Physical therapy, occupational therapy

REVIEW QUESTIONS

1. A 48-year-old man comes to the physician for follow-up examination. He was involved in a motor vehicle accident 3 months ago. Since then, he has been using a wheelchair due to paraparesis. Physical exam shows spasticity and 4+ deep tendon reflexes in the lower extremities. Pain and temperature sensation are lost in both legs; however proprioception and vibration sensation are intact. Physical examination of upper extremities is unremarkable. What is the most likely diagnosis?

   - **The most likely diagnosis is anterior cord syndrome.**
   - This patient has been using a wheelchair due to paraparesis after he was involved in a motor vehicle accident.
   - Physical examination shows spasticity and 4+ deep tendon reflexes in the lower extremities. These findings indicate an UMN lesion and damage to the lateral corticospinal tracts.
   - Pain and temperature sensation are also lost in the legs suggesting damage to the lateral spinothalamic tracts.
   - Proprioception and vibration sensation are intact which means the dorsal columns are intact.
   - Damage to all the major tracts except for the dorsal columns suggests the diagnosis of anterior cord syndrome. This is most commonly caused by the injury of the anterior spinal artery.

2. A 37-year-old woman is brought to the emergency department after accidentally burning her hand. She did not feel the heat or pain from the burn. Physical exam shows loss of pain and temperature sensation along with flaccid weakness and 1+ deep tendon reflexes in both upper extremities. Physical examination of the lower extremities is unremarkable. What is the most likely diagnosis?

   - **The most likely diagnosis is central cord syndrome.**
   - This woman burned her hand but she did not feel the heat or pain from the burn.
   - Physical examination shows loss of pain and temperature sensation only in the upper extremities, suggesting injury to the spinothalamic fibers in the anterior white commissure.
   - Additionally, there is flaccid weakness and hypoactive deep tendon reflexes in the upper extremities indicating injury to the ventral horns at the cervical cord level.

REVIEW QUESTIONS

3. A 52-year-old man is brought to the emergency department by his partner 2-days after being in a motor vehicle accident. Physical examination shows spastic paresis of the right lower extremity with 4+ deep tendon reflexes. There is loss of vibration sensation and proprioception on the right leg. Pain and temperature sensation are lost in the left lower extremity below the level of inguinal ligament. What is the most likely diagnosis in this patient?

- **The most likely diagnosis is Brown-Sequard syndrome.**
- This man presents with neurological deficits shortly after being involved in a motorcycle accident.
- Physical examination shows spastic paresis of the right lower extremity with 4+ deep tendon reflexes. These findings indicate an upper motor neuron lesion and damage of the corticospinal tract.
- There is loss of vibration sensation and proprioception on the right leg, suggesting damage to the dorsal columns.
- Pain and temperature sensation are lost in the left lower extremity below the level of inguinal ligament. This clue points to damage to the spinothalamic tract.
- All of these neurological deficits within the context of trauma suggest the diagnosis of Brown-Sequard syndrome.
- In Brown-Sequard syndrome, the pain and temperature sensation are lost 1-2 levels below the lesion.
- Inguinal ligament coincides with the L1 dermatome. The spinal cord segments 1 to 2 levels above L1 will be T11 or T12. Therefore, the patient has Brown-Sequard syndrome with right T11/12 segment trans-section.

4. A 67-year-old women is brought to the emergency department by her daughter because of spastic paralysis of both lower extremities for the last 3 days. The patient also admits to recently experiencing incontinence more frequently. Physical examination shows she has loss of pain and temperature sensation in both lower extremities; however, her vibration sense and proprioception are intact bilaterally. The patient is sent for an MRI which shows a herniated vertebral disc compressing a nearby artery. Based on this patient's presentation, which of the following spinal tracts are most likely damaged?

   A. Dorsal columns and lateral spinothalamic tract
   B. Lateral spinothalamic and corticospinal tracts
   C. Anterior horn neurons and spinothalamic tract
   D. Lateral spinothalamic tract and cervical sympathetics

- **The correct answer is option B.**
- This elderly woman presents with spastic paralysis of both lower extremities, incontinence, and loss of pain and temperature sensation in both lower extremities.
- She has her vibration sense and proprioception intact bilaterally. Based on these features, she is experiencing anterior cord syndrome.
- This is confirmed by the MRI showing a herniated lumbar disc which is most likely compressing the anterior spinal artery.
- Anterior spinal injury damages the lateral corticospinal tracts causing bilateral spastic paralysis at and below the lesion level. It damages the lateral spinothalamic tracts causing bilateral loss of pain and temperature sensation. It also damages the autonomic tracts descending to the sacral cord causing incontinence. It spares the dorsal column which is why there is intact vibration sense and proprioception.
- Option A, dorsal columns and lateral spinothalamic tract, and option D, lateral spinothalamic tract and cervical sympathetics, are incorrect because these tracts would be injured in Brown-Sequard syndrome. In anterior cord syndrome the dorsal columns and cervical sympathetics are not damaged.
- Option C, anterior horn neurons and spinothalamic tract, is incorrect because these would be injured in central cord syndrome. In anterior cord syndrome the anterior horn neurons are not damaged.

Neurology | Section 16: Cauda Equina Syndrome, Syringomyelia & Transverse Myelitis

I. Cauda Equina Syndrome: Definition
   A. Compression of the spinal nerve roots in the lumbar and sacral regions of the spinal canal

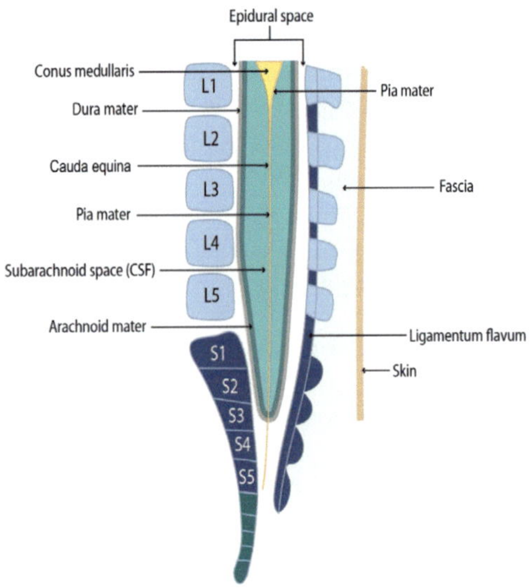

FIGURE 13.1.82 - Spinal Canal and Cauda Equina

II. Cauda Equina Syndrome: Etiology
   A. Vertebral disc herniation
   B. Epidural abscess
   C. Epidural tumor
   D. Lumbar spine spondylosis

III. Cauda Equina Syndrome: Clinical Features
   A. Back pain with unilateral/bilateral leg pain
   B. Loss of sensory and motor function in lower extremities (e.g. weakness of plantar flexion, absent DTRs)
   C. Saddle anesthesia
   D. Bladder and bowel dysfunction

IV. Cauda Equina Syndrome: Diagnosis and Management
   A. Diagnosis
      1. MRI (imaging test of choice)
   B. Management
      1. Emergent surgical decompression

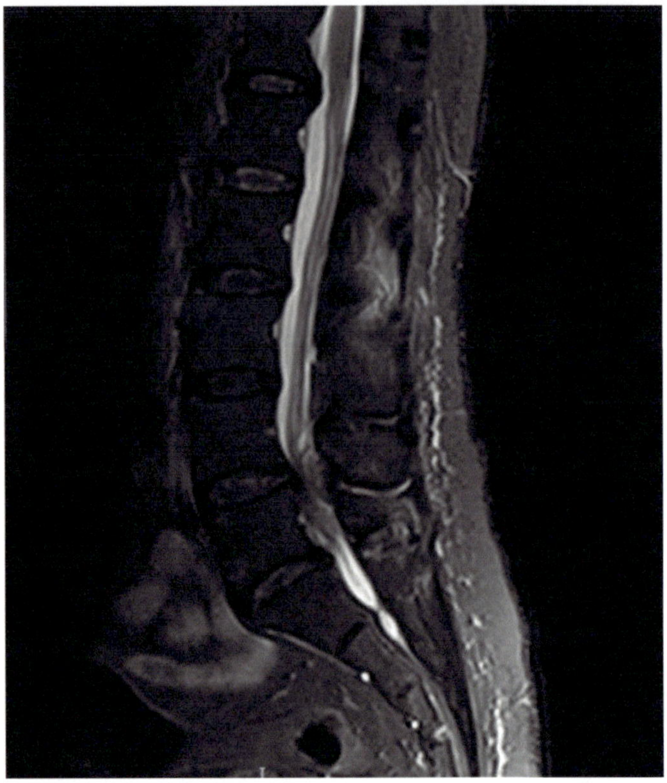

FIGURE 13.1.83 - MRI of Lumbosacral Spine

V. Syringomyelia: Definition
   A. Fluid-filled cavity within the spinal cord that damages adjacent spinal tracts and structures
   B. Dilation of the central canal or separate cavity within the parenchyma
   C. Most often affects cervical or thoracic cord (C2-T9)

VI. Syringomyelia: Etiology
   A. Chiari malformation type I (most common)
   B. Neoplasms (e.g. ependymoma)
   C. Spinal trauma
   D. Infections
   E. Inflammation (e.g. transverse myelitis)

VII. Syringomyelia: Clinical Features
   A. May be asymptomatic
   B. Damage of spinothalamic fibers in anterior white commissure
      1. Bilateral loss of pain and temperature sensation over the upper back, neck, and arms ("cape-like" distribution)
   C. Compressing anterior horn cells
      1. LMN lesion: bilateral flaccid weakness, diminished DTRs at lesion level

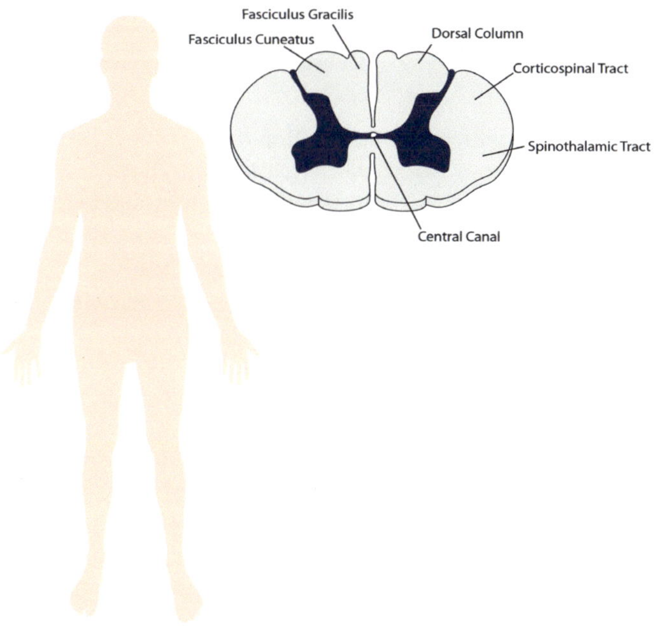

FIGURE 13.1.84- Cross Section of the Spinal Cord with a Human Outline

VIII. Syringomyelia: Diagnosis and Management
   A. Diagnosis
      1. MRI: fluid-filled lesion
   B. Management
      1. Surgical decompression, shunt placement

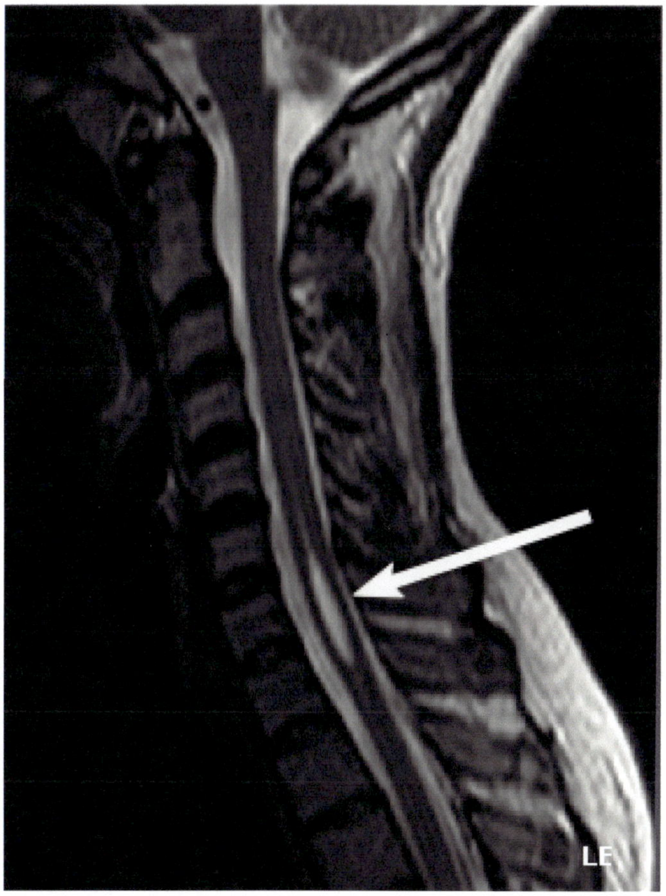

FIGURE 13.1.85 - Syringomyelia

IX. Transverse Myelitis: Definition
   A. Acute inflammation of spinal cord segment(s)
   B. Most commonly affects the thoracic cord
   C. May be primary or secondary (disease-associated)

X. Transverse Myelitis: Etiology
   A. Idiopathic
   B. Infections: viral (e.g. enteroviruses), bacterial (e.g. *Mycoplasma*)
   C. CNS disorders: multiple sclerosis
   D. Systemic inflammatory autoimmune disorders: sarcoidosis, SLE, Sjogren's syndrome

XI. Transverse Myelitis: Clinical Features
   A. Acute/subacute onset
   B. Bilateral weakness and altered sensation (e.g. pain, paresthesia)
   C. Autonomic dysfunction (e.g. bowel and bladder incontinence)
   D. On neurologic examination: sensory level is identified

XII. Transverse Myelitis: Diagnosis
   A. MRI with/without gadolinium: gadolinium-enhancing signal abnormality over one or more segments of spinal cord
   B. Lumbar puncture and CSF analysis: moderate pleocytosis, elevated protein, normal glucose

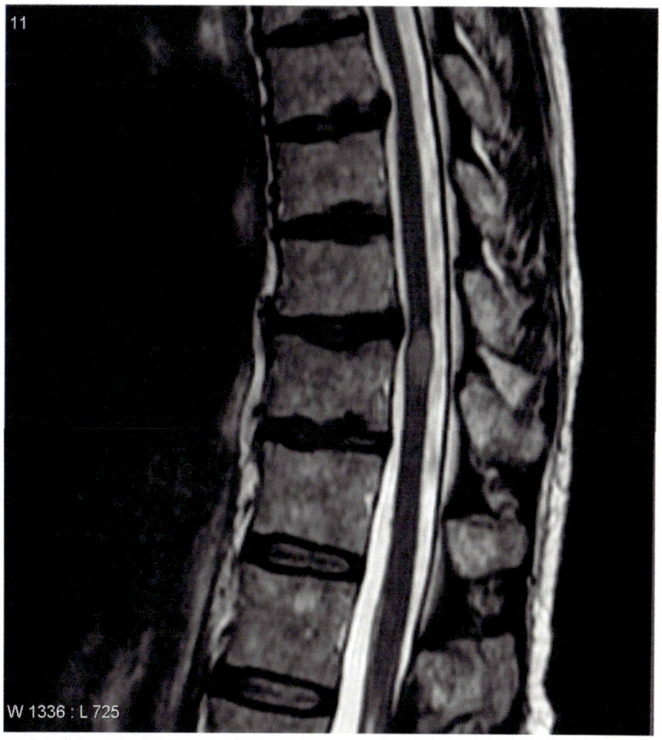

FIGURE 13.1.86 - Spinal MRI: Transverse Myelitis

XIII. Transverse Myelitis: Management
   A. High-dose intravenous glucocorticoids
   B. Plasma exchange
   C. Prognosis: partial recovery is expected in idiopathic TM within three months

REVIEW QUESTIONS

1. A 71-year-old woman is brought to the emergency room because of urinary and fecal incontinence for the past week. She also reports unintentional weight loss and severe back pain during this time. Physical examination shows weakness of the lower extremities with 1+ deep tendon reflexes. Perineal anesthesia is noted on the sensory examination. What is the best next step in management of this patient?

    - **The best next step in management of this patient is an urgent MRI of the lumbosacral spine.**
    - This elderly woman presents with urinary and fecal incontinence along with severe back pain for the past week.
    - Physical exam shows weakness of the lower extremities with 1+ deep tendon reflexes.
    - Perineal anesthesia is noted on the sensory examination.
    - Urinary and fecal incontinence, back pain, lower extremity weakness, and saddle anesthesia raise suspicion for cauda equina syndrome.
    - Given the history of unintentional weight loss, cauda equina syndrome may be secondary to malignancy.

2. A 35-year-old woman comes to the physician because of worsening urinary and fecal incontinence for the past month. She has a medical history of poorly controlled multiple sclerosis. Vital signs include temperature of 96.8° F (36° C), blood pressure of 110/75 mmHg, heart rate of 88 beats/min, and respiratory rate of 16 breaths/min. Physical examination shows loss of vibration, proprioception, pain, and temperature sensation bilaterally below the level of nipples. Spastic weakness with 3+ deep tendon reflexes are noted in the lower extremities. The upper extremities are unremarkable. MRI with gadolinium enhancement shows enhanced signals at the T4 spinal cord segment. CSF analysis after lumbar puncture shows 30 lymphocytes/mm^3, 50 mg/dL protein, and 60 mg/dL glucose. Which of the following is the most likely diagnosis in this patient?

    A. Transverse myelitis
    B. Amyotrophic lateral sclerosis
    C. Anterior cord syndrome
    D. Central cord syndrome

    - **The correct answer is option A.**
    - This young woman with poorly controlled multiple sclerosis presents with urinary and fecal incontinence for the past month.
    - Physical examination shows loss of vibration, proprioception, pain, and temperature sensation bilaterally below the level of nipples.
    - Below the level of the nipple all sensations are impaired suggesting damage to both dorsal columns and spinothalamic tracts.
    - Spastic weakness with 3+ deep tendon reflexes are noted in the lower extremities indicating damage to the corticospinal tracts.
    - MRI with gadolinium enhancement shows enhanced signals at the T4 spinal cord segment.
    - CSF analysis is significant for mild pleocytosis evidenced by 30 lymphocytes/mm^3 and mildly increased protein with the level of 50 mg/dL.
    - All of these findings point to the diagnosis of transverse myelitis.
    - Transverse myelitis is even more likely given this patient's history of multiple sclerosis.
    - Option B is incorrect because amyotrophic lateral sclerosis is not characterized by sensory disturbances. Additionally, it usually presents with flaccid weakness in the upper extremities which is absent in this patient.
    - Option C is incorrect because anterior cord syndrome damages all major tracts except the dorsal column system. This patient has lost vibration and proprioception indicating dorsal column damage, therefore, anterior cord syndrome is excluded.
    - Option D is incorrect because central cord syndrome is characterized by loss of pain and temperature and the flaccid weakness at the level of the lesions. In addition to pain and temperature sensation, this patient has also lost vibration and proprioception, and she has spastic, rather than flaccid, weakness.

Neurology | Section 17: Poliomyelitis, Amyotrophic Lateral Sclerosis & Horner Syndrome

I. Poliomyelitis: Definition
   A. Acute infection that damages anterior horn cells of spinal cord and lower motor neurons of brainstem
   B. The responsible pathogen is poliovirus (neurotropic enterovirus)

II. Poliomyelitis: Clinical Features
   A. LMN lesion: acute flaccid weakness, absent DTRs
   B. Bulbar involvement: respiratory and cardiovascular failure
   C. Sensation is intact
   D. Aseptic meningitis
      1. Fever, nausea, headache, nuchal rigidity

III. Poliomyelitis: Diagnosis and Management
   A. Clinical findings are suggestive
   B. Lumbar puncture and CSF analysis: moderate pleocytosis, elevated protein
   C. Isolation of virus from stool (golden standard), CSF PCR
   D. Management: supportive
      1. Pain management, physical therapy, mechanical ventilation in case of respiratory failure

IV. Amyotrophic Lateral Sclerosis: Definition
   A. Lou Gehrig disease
   B. Progressive neurodegenerative disorder
   C. Both UMN and LMN deficits

V. Amyotrophic Lateral Sclerosis: Clinical Features
   A. Typical presentation: asymmetric limb weakness
   B. UMN lesion
      1. Spasticity
      2. Exaggerated DTRs (hyperreflexia)
      3. Pseudobulbar palsy: dysarthria, dysphagia, increased or normal gag reflex

VI. Amyotrophic Lateral Sclerosis: Clinical Features
   A. LMN lesion
      1. Flaccid weakness
      2. Fasciculations
      3. Muscle atrophy
      4. Bulbar palsy: dysarthria, dysphagia, absent gag reflex
   B. Respiratory failure is the main cause of death

VII. Amyotrophic Lateral Sclerosis: Diagnosis
   A. Diagnosis is primarily clinical
   B. Electrodiagnostic studies
      1. Electromyography (EMG): acute and chronic denervation
      2. Nerve conduction studies: normal
   C. Neuroimaging (MRI): exclude other diagnoses

VIII. Amyotrophic Lateral Sclerosis: Management
   A. Riluzole
      1. Prolongs survival and slows disease progression
      2. Side effects: dizziness, weight loss, asthenia, ↑ liver enzymes

IX. Horner Syndrome: Definition
   A. Oculosympathetic paresis
   B. Lesion along the sympathetic pathway that supplies head, neck, and eye

X. Horner Syndrome: Etiology
   A. Wallenberg syndrome (lateral medullary infarction)
   B. Cervical cord trauma
   C. Pancoast tumor
   D. Carotid artery dissection
   E. Carotid endarterectomy

The Oculosympathetic Pathway

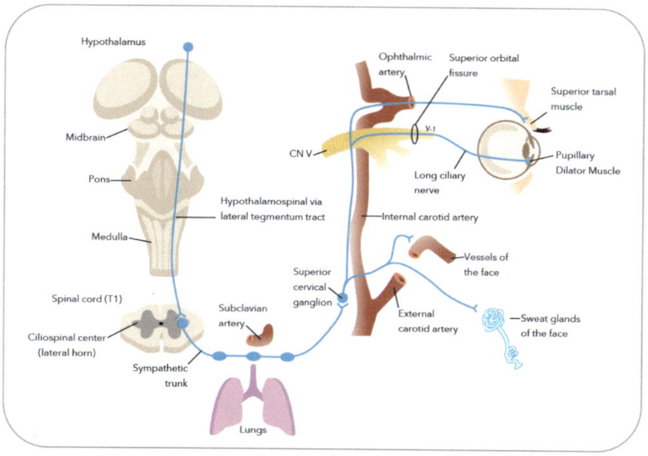

FIGURE 13.1.87 - Oculosympathetic Pathway

XI. Horner Syndrome: Clinical Features
   A. Ipsilateral miosis
   B. Ipsilateral ptosis (paralysis of Muller's muscle)
   C. Ipsilateral anhidrosis (central / preganglionic lesions)

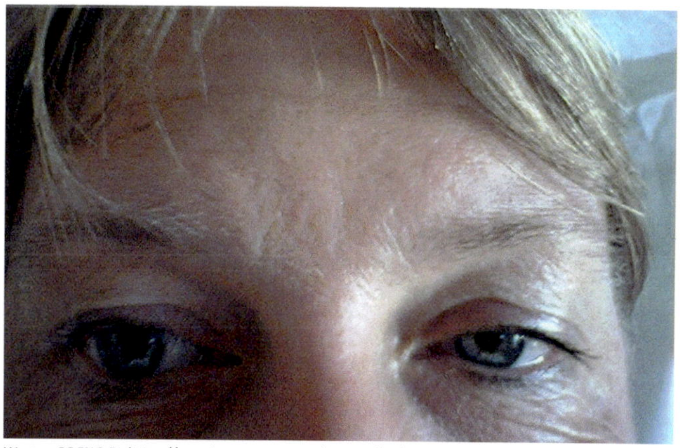

FIGURE 13.1.88 - Miosis and Ptosis in a Patient with Horner Syndrome

XII. Horner Syndrome: Diagnosis and Management
   A. Cocaine or apraclonidine eye drops to confirm the diagnosis
      1. Cocaine: anisocoria of ≥ 1 mm is confirmatory
      2. Apraclonidine: reversal anisocoria is confirmatory
   B. Hydroxyamphetamine eye drops for localizing the lesion
      1. Anisocoria of ≥ 1 mm is positive for postganglionic lesion
   C. Neuroimaging (MRI)
   D. Management: treat underlying cause

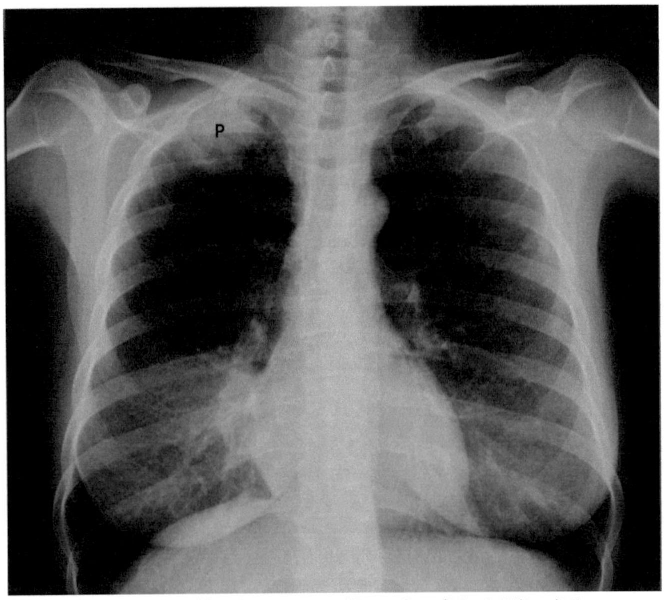

FIGURE 13.1.89 - Pancoast Tumor on Chest X-Ray

REVIEW QUESTIONS

1. A 5-year-old boy is brought to the emergency department by his parents because of fevers and acute weakness for the past 2 days. He vomited three times en route to the hospital. He is not vaccinated due to parental beliefs. Physical examination shows flaccid weakness in the lower extremities along with positive Kernig and Brudzinski signs. What is the most likely diagnosis in this patient?

   - **The most likely diagnosis in this patient is poliomyelitis.**
   - This young boy presents with high fever, vomiting, and weakness.
   - Physical exam shows flaccid weakness of lower extremities along with positive Kernig and Brudzinski signs.
   - The acute onset flaccid weakness and the signs of meningitis raise strong suspicion for poliomyelitis.
   - Poliomyelitis is more likely given he is not vaccinated.

2. A 67-year-old man comes to the physician due to progressively worsening hand weakness for the past 6 months. Physical examination shows flaccid weakness along with 1+ deep tendon reflexes in both upper extremities. Spastic weakness and 4+ deep tendon reflexes are noted in both lower extremities. Sensation is intact throughout the body. What is the best pharmacologic management option for this patient?

   - **The best pharmacologic management option for this patient is riluzole which slows down the neuronal degeneration and prolongs survival.**
   - This elderly man presents with progressively worsening hand weakness for the past 6 months.
   - Physical examination shows flaccid weakness along with 1+ deep tendon reflexes in both upper extremities indicating damage to the ventral horns of the spinal cord, a LMN lesion.
   - Spastic weakness and 4+ deep tendon reflexes are noted in both lower extremities suggesting damage to the corticospinal tracts, a UMN lesion.
   - Sensation is intact throughout the body.
   - Lower motor neuron signs in the upper extremities, upper motor neuron signs in lower extremities, and intact sensation are consistent with the diagnosis of amyotrophic lateral sclerosis.

REVIEW QUESTIONS

3. A 68-year-old man comes to the physician due to a droopy eyelid for the past 4 months. He noticed he cannot properly open his left eye, and his left pupil is smaller than the right one. When he plays football with his grandchildren, the left side of his face does not sweat. He also has severe shoulder pain which is worse at night. The patient has been smoking 2.5 packs of cigarettes per day for the past 50 years. Physical examination is otherwise normal. Which underlying condition most likely accounts for this patient's current complaints?

- **Given this patient's shoulder pain and extensive smoking history, the most likely underlying condition that accounts for this patient's Horner syndrome is Pancoast tumor.**
- This elderly man reports a droopy eyelid for the past 4 months.
- This finding is known as ptosis.
- He also noticed that his left pupil is smaller than the right one.
- So he has left-sided miosis and resultant anisocoria.
- When he plays football with his grandchildren, the left side of his face does not sweat.
- This sign is consistent with anhidrosis.
- Ptosis, miosis, and anhidrosis are the classic signs of Horner syndrome.
- The patient also complains of severe shoulder pain which is worse at night.
- He has been smoking 2.5 packs of cigarettes per day for the past 50 years.
- Pancoast tumor is a superior sulcus tumor in the lung apex which can compress the stellate ganglion, disrupt the sympathetic fibers, and cause a secondary Horner syndrome.

4. An 11-year-old boy is brought by his parents to the emergency department because of acute onset of fever, nausea, and headache. His parents recently immigrated and are unable to speak fluent English. Physical examination shows diffuse flaccid weakness as well as diminished deep tendon reflexes bilaterally. There is also significant nuchal rigidity. When the patient's neck is flexed by the physician, the patient's hips and knees flex in response. A complete blood count shows all values within normal limits. Based on the most likely diagnosis, what is the next best step in the management of this patient?

   A. Broad spectrum antibiotics
   B. Chest X-ray
   C. Lumbar puncture
   D. Electromyography

- **The correct answer is option C.**
- This 11-year old male presents with acute onset fever, nausea, headache, nuchal rigidity, flaccid weakness, and diminished deep tendon reflexes.
- He recently immigrated and may not have received all his childhood vaccinations.
- A positive Kernig sign indicates inflammation of the meninges, concerning for meningitis.
- Since the CBC is within normal limits and not showing leukocytosis, we can assume the meningitis is not bacterial in nature.
- The presentation of acute onset of aseptic meningitis with headache, fever, nausea, and nuchal rigidity along with unknown vaccination status is consistent with poliomyelitis.
- In the management of suspected meningitis or poliomyelitis, a lumbar puncture with CSF analysis is often performed first.
- Option A is incorrect because broad spectrum antibiotics are not used in the management of poliomyelitis since the etiology is viral.
- Option B is incorrect because a chest X-ray could be used in the management of Horner Syndrome if a pancoast tumor is suspected, not in poliomyelitis.
- Option D is incorrect because electromyography could be used in the diagnosis and management of amyotrophic lateral sclerosis, not poliomyelitis.

Neurology | Section 18: Seizures: Causes, Types, and Workup

I. Seizures: General Information
   A. Abnormal excessive neuronal electrical discharges from cortical regions of the brain
   B. Two general types: partial and generalized seizures; based on whether one or both hemispheres were involved

II. Seizures: Causes
   A. Inducing causes: provoked seizures
      1. Neurological: brain tumors, strokes, brain bleeds, structural brain abnormalities, CNS infections
      2. Others
         a) Internal: strong emotional stimuli, alkalosis, drugs, alcohol, high fever
         b) External: loud noises, flashing lights, sleep deprivation
   B. Causes by age
      1. Neonates: idiopathic, congenital, genetic, perinatal injury, metabolic
      2. Infants/children: idiopathic, fever, trauma, infections
      3. Adolescents: illicit substance use (drug intoxication/withdrawal)
      4. Adults: alcoholism (alcohol withdrawal), illicit substance use
      5. Older adults (> 35 years): stroke, brain tumor, trauma, metabolic

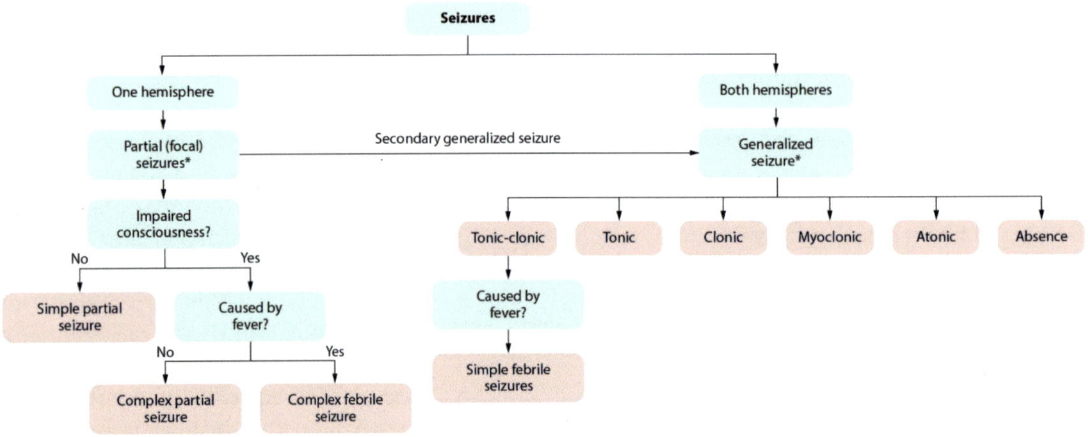

FIGURE 13.1.90 - Types of Seizures

Type	Definition	Key Features
Simple partial seizure	- Seizures from one hemisphere - Awareness is intact	- Motor: Jacksonian March (rhythmic twitching spreading along body parts) - Sensory and psychiatric: tingling, hallucinations, déjà vu, fear - Postictal: Todd's paralysis: affected muscles (limbs or facial muscles) are paralyzed up to 24 hours after
Complex partial seizure	- Seizures from one hemisphere (usually temporal lobe) - Awareness is impaired	- Automatisms (lip-smacking, chewing movements, or picking at clothing) - Aura (smell, visual, taste, and hearing) - Postictal: amnesia, aphasia (speech arrest) or nonsensical speech
Generalized tonic-clonic	- Abnormal electrical activity involving both hemispheres - Awareness is impaired	- Alternating tonic (muscle contraction) and clonic (muscle twitching) phases - Other: tongue-biting, incontinence, vomiting, cyanosis, apnea - Postictal: confusion, amnesia, muscle flaccidity
Absence or "petit mal seizures"	- Occurs in childhood or early adolescence - Awareness is impaired	- Lasts for 3-30 seconds - Staring into space - Rapid gain of consciousness - Many times (100s) a day

TABLE 13.1.9 - Types of Seizures

Type	Definition	Key Features
Atonic or "drop" seizures	- Generalized motor seizure characterized by loss of muscle tone - "Akinetic seizures"	- Sudden loss of muscle strength → fall or "drop" to the floor - Brief loss of consciousness - No postictal phase
Myoclonic seizures	- Associated with seizure syndromes - Affect 3-12 month old infants/children (Lennox-Gastaut syndrome, infant spasms) or adolescents (juvenile myoclonic epilepsy)	- Sudden jerk with muscle twitching - Brief loss of consciousness - No postictal phase
Febrile seizures	- Triggered by high grade fever > 38° C (100.4° F) - Most common in children of 6 months up to 5 years of age	- Simple febrile seizures: few seconds to 15 minutes; do not recur within 24 hours - Complex febrile seizures: > 15 minutes; recurs within 24 hours of the first seizure - Postictal: rapid return to normal

TABLE 13.1.10 - Types of Seizures

C. Status epilepticus
   1. Continuous seizure for ≥ 5 mins or ≥ 2 seizures without regaining of consciousness in between the episodes
   2. A medical emergency
   3. Can lead to cerebral edema, cortical laminar necrosis, rhabdomyolysis, and cardiovascular collapse

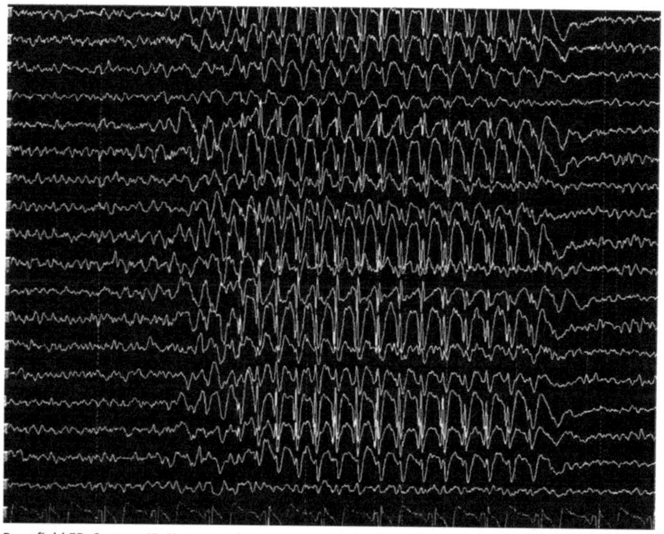

FIGURE 13.1.91 - EEG: Generalized 3 Hz Spike-Wave Discharge in Absence Seizures

III. Seizures: Workup
   A. General workup
      1. Confirm seizure diagnosis
      2. Look for underlying condition
   B. Confirm seizure diagnosis
      1. History: from patients and bystanders; recollection of the incident, presence of an aura; possible inducing factors (e.g. sleep deprivation, medications)
      2. Obtain an EEG: look for epileptiform discharges
      3. Seizure-specific EEG findings: absence (3-Hz-spike-wave)
   C. Look for underlying condition
      1. ECG: exclude arrhythmias, cardiogenic causes
      2. Brain CT/MRI: look for structural causes (e.g. AVM); brain lesions
      3. Blood work: CBC, BMP, ESR, LFTs, toxicology screen
      4. CSF analysis: exclude CNS infection
      5. Urine drug test
   D. Status epilepticus
      1. Diagnosis is mostly clinical
      2. Diagnostic criteria
         a) Continuous seizure for ≥ 5 mins or
         b) ≥ 2 seizures without the regain of consciousness in between the episodes

REVIEW QUESTIONS

1. A 40-year-old man is brought to the hospital via ambulance. He was found unconscious on the street. During transit to the hospital he began seizing. The medics report that the seizure has been going on for at least 5 minutes. After administration of IV lorazepam, the seizure stops. This patient is at risk of developing what neurological complication?

    - **This patient is at risk of developing cerebral edema and cortical laminar necrosis.**
    - This patient has been seizing for at least 5 minutes and is in status epilepticus.
    - Patients with status epilepticus are at risk of developing neurological complications such as cerebral edema and cortical laminar necrosis due to prolonged brain hypoxia.
    - Other important complications include rhabdomyolysis and cardiovascular collapse.

2. A 10-year-old boy is brought to the physician by his mother because of multiple episodes of staring blankly. She says these episodes last for several minutes and he is not responsive during them. She does not recall any precipitating factors. Ten days ago she witnessed one of his episodes where he just stared into space while picking continuously at his clothes. She had also noticed mild facial grimacing during the episode. He does not remember these episodes but recalls smelling a strange smell prior to the episode and feels confused and lethargic after. Physical and neurological exams show no abnormalities. What is the most likely diagnosis of this patient?

    A. Simple partial seizure
    B. Absence seizure
    C. Complex partial seizure
    D. Myoclonic seizure
    E. Atonic seizure

    - **The correct answer is option C.**
    - This 10-year-old boy is brought in because of multiple episodes of staring. His staring episodes are accompanied by automatisms such as lip smacking, facial grimacing, picking at his clothes, and an olfactory aura where he smells something strange. He does not remember the episodes and feels confused and lethargic after. All these are features of complex partial seizure.
    - Complex partial seizures are seizures arising from one hemisphere, usually temporal lobe where the awareness is impaired. Key features of this type include automatisms such as lip-smacking, chewing movements, or picking at clothing. Auras such as smell, visual, taste, and hearing auras may also be present like we saw in our patient. In the postictal period, patients may experience some amnesia, aphasia or speech arrest, or nonsensical speech
    - Option A is incorrect because, even though patients can present with auras, patients do not lose their consciousness during the episodes.
    - Option B is incorrect because these episodes last for a few seconds and not several minutes like we see in this patient. Absence seizures also lack a postictal phase, patients do not experience confusion or lethargy after the episode, and auras are not present.
    - Option D is incorrect because myoclonic seizures are characterized by brief jerking movements which are absent in this patient.
    - Option E is incorrect because in atonic seizures, patients briefly lose their muscle tone which leads to head nodding or dropping to the floor during the episodes, both of which are absent in this patient.

Neurology | Section 19: Seizures: Differential Diagnosis and Management

Condition	Etiology	Key Features
Psychogenic or "pseudoseizures"	- Psychiatric origin	- Absence of tongue biting, urinary, and fecal incontinence; closed eyes and side-to-side movement during the episode - No abnormal activity on EEG
Syncope	- Vasovagal syncope - Cardiogenic - Orthostatic hypotension - Carotid sinus syndrome	- Triggers such as positional changes (orthostatic), emotional stimulus (vasovagal), pressure on the carotid sinus (carotid sinus syndrome) - Abnormal ECG findings such as complete AV block (Stokes-Adams attack)
Breath-holding spells	- Triggered by strong emotions (e.g. anger, pain)	- Children 6 months to 6 years - Can mimic seizure; children will present with muscle stiffness and jerks - Apnea → loss of consciousness with cyanosis and pallor
Inattentive staring spells	- Normal inattention due to boredom	- Mostly occurs during boring activities - Absence of automatisms - Response to vocal or tactile stimulus
Psychological conditions	- Panic attacks - Psychogenic hyperventilation	- Symptoms include tachycardia, hyperventilation, diaphoresis, and shortness of breath

TABLE 13.1.11 - Differential Diagnosis of Seizures

I. Seizures: Management
   A. General management
      1. Remove objects around the patient to avoid self-injury
      2. Establish and maintain airway, breathing and circulation by providing oxygen and start IV fluids
      3. Monitor vitals (temperature, blood pressure, oxygen saturation)
   B. 1st seizure; patients with no history of epilepsy
      1. Low risk of recurrence with a normal EEG
      2. Anticonvulsant therapy not required
      3. If EEG or brain MRI are abnormal start pharmacotherapy (antiepileptics)
      4. Eliminating underlying cause is usually sufficient
   C. Febrile seizures
      1. Uncomplicated: no treatment required; spontaneously resolve in < 5 mins
      2. Complicated (≥ 5 mins) or complex febrile seizures: abortive therapy with IV benzodiazepines (lorazepam) with buccal/intranasal benzodiazepines as an alternative
      3. Follow-up with antipyretic treatment (e.g. acetaminophen, NSAIDs)
   D. Recurrent focal seizures of unknown cause
      1. 1st line: lamotrigine, phenytoin, carbamazepine; phenobarbital (children)
   E. Recurrent generalized seizures of unknown cause
      1. Tonic-clonic
         a) 1st line: valproate, lamotrigine; phenobarbital for children
         b) 2nd line: carbamazepine
      2. Absence seizures (typical): ethosuximide, valproate
      3. All others (myoclonic, atypical absence)
         a) 1st line: valproate, lamotrigine
         a. Patients with a known history of epilepsy
      4. Seizure most likely due to medication non compliance
      5. A loading dose of their medications should be administered followed by maintenance of regular dosage
      6. Treatment principle: if seizures persist, increase the dose; if toxicities occur, add another antiepileptic instead
      7. Medication can be tapered down after being 2 years seizure-free
   F. Other medical therapies
      1. Vagus nerve stimulation: device implanted under the skin in the chest region; provides impulses through the course of the vagus nerve to the brain
      2. Surgery: resecting the problematic part (e.g. anterior temporal lobectomy treat intractable temporal lobe seizures, hemispherectomy)
   G. Status epilepticus
      1. Rapid neurological assessment
      2. Supportive treatment (e.g. IV access, O_2, glucose, thiamine)
      3. Pharmacological intervention
   H. Pharmacological intervention
      1. IV benzodiazepines (1st line): lorazepam or diazepam; rectal diazepam, buccal or intranasal lorazepam/midazolam
      2. No response after 1 minute: additional dose of benzodiazepines
      3. No response: continuous antiepileptic drug along with an anesthetic (e.g. thiopental, propofol)
      4. Intubation and admission to the ICU

REVIEW QUESTIONS

1. A 16-year-old girl is admitted to the hospital because of multiple episodes of loss of consciousness and jerking body movements. She does not recall the episodes and denies the presence of any aura. Laboratory studies are unremarkable. During her hospitalization she is placed on continuous EEG. She experiences another episode where the nurse noted the patient's eyes rolling backward and her body swinging side-to-side before falling to the ground. She also noted repetitive violent jerking of all limbs. The EEG shows no indication of a seizure during the event. The patient has never experienced tongue biting nor fecal or urinary incontinence during the episodes. What is the most likely cause of this patient's condition?
   - **The most likely cause of this patient's condition is pseudo or psychogenic seizures.**
   - This 16-year-old girl is admitted to the hospital because of multiple episodes of loss of consciousness and jerking body movements that raise suspicion of seizures.
   - During her hospitalization, side-to-side body movement, lack of tongue biting, fecal, or urinary incontinence during the episode make pseudo or psychogenic seizures more likely even the intensity of these episodes with normal EEG.

2. A 5-year-old girl is brought to the emergency department via ambulance with her parents because of a seizure. The seizure has been ongoing for 5 minutes. Her parents state that she has been having intermittent high fevers because of a respiratory tract infection. Her temperature is 103.5° F (39.7° C). What is the best next step in management?
   - **The next best step is IV lorazepam.**
   - This child with a seizure and very high fever is most likely having a febrile seizure.
   - She has been seizing for 5 minutes, and therefore, requires abortive therapy with intravenous lorazepam as a treatment of choice.
   - Febrile seizures are usually uncomplicated and resolve within a few minutes on their own. However, febrile seizures that occur for 5 minutes or more and complex febrile seizures require abortive therapy.
   - After administration of IV benzodiazepines, antipyretic therapy with an NSAID or acetaminophen is required.

3. A 25-year-old man with a history of epilepsy is brought to the emergency department via ambulance because he started seizing in his workplace 20 minutes prior. When he arrived to the hospital his jerky movements had stopped, but he has remained unresponsive. While the physician was performing the physical exmination his arms and legs started to jerk again. What is the best next step in management?
   - **The next best step is to perform the ABCs and administer IV benzodiazepines.**
   - This patient was brought in because of a seizure. He has now had two seizures without regaining consciousness in between.
   - His past medical history is significant for epilepsy.
   - He is experiencing status epilepticus, a life-threatening medical emergency.
   - After ensuring adequate airway, breathing, and circulation, intravenous benzodiazepines should be administered to abort the seizure activity.

REVIEW QUESTIONS

4. A 7-year-old boy is brought to the emergency department by his parents because of confusion and amnesia after a sudden loss of consciousness followed by generalized muscle contractions and twitching. The patient's mother stated that his eyes seemed to roll backward as he was shaking just like the last three times this happened. This episode lasted roughly 3 minutes. Upon closer inspection it is noted that the patient has bitten the side of his tongue and urinated on himself. Vital signs include a temperature of 98.8° F (37.1° C), heart rate of 125 bpm, respiratory rate of 22 bpm, blood pressure of 140/100 mmHg, and O_2 saturation at 96%. Which of the following is the best next step in management?

    A. Lamotrigine
    B. Lorazepam
    C. Ethosuximide
    D. Phenobarbital

- **The correct answer is option D.**
- This child presents with confusion and amnesia after sudden loss of consciousness associated with muscle contractions and twitching.
- This presentation suggests a tonic-clonic seizure with the muscle contractions representing the tonic phase and muscle twitching representing the clonic phase. The current confusion and amnesia represents the post-ictal phase of the seizure.
- Additional support for the diagnosis of tonic-clonic seizure includes rotated eyes and bladder incontinence.
- Vital signs show the expected increased sympathetic tone in the form of tachycardia and hypertension.
- Often during a seizure breathing patterns are disrupted, so afterwards a lower saturation and increased breathing is expected.
- Since this is a child having recurrent tonic-clonic seizures with the cause unknown, the best medical management would be phenobarbital.
- Option A is incorrect because even though lamotrigine is first line for recurrent tonic-clonic seizures, phenobarbital is first line for children.
- Option B is incorrect because benzodiazepines are indicated in the management of complicated febrile seizures, not recurrent tonic-clonic seizures, and this child does not have a fever.
- Option C is incorrect because ethosuximide is indicated in the management of typical absence seizures not recurrent tonic-clonic seizures.

Neurology | Section 20: Aphasia and Neglect

I. Aphasia: Definition
  A. Aphasia is an acquired abnormality of language, typically with difficulties in comprehension or expression
    1. Usually due to focal brain lesion

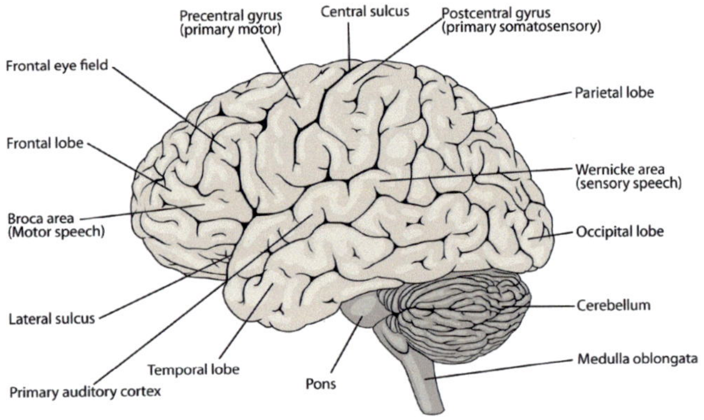

FIGURE 13.1.92 - Anatomy of the Brain

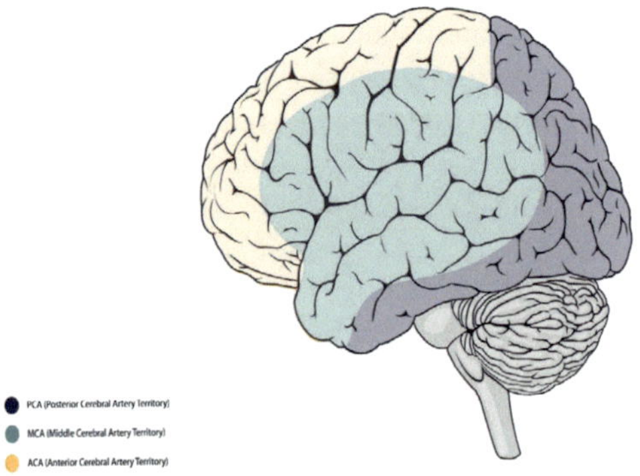

FIGURE 13.1.93 - Blood Supply to Different Areas of the Brain

II. Broca's Aphasia
  A. Problem of language production with impaired repetition
  B. Will have normal comprehension
  C. Patients usually aware of deficit and are frustrated by it
  D. Broca's area: frontal lobe (dominant hemisphere)
    1. Typically involves strokes involving superior division of the MCA
    2. Can be associated with other symptoms: contralateral weakness of face and arm

III. Wernicke's Aphasia
  A. Problem with language comprehension with impaired repetition
  B. Speech is fluent but nonsensical ("word salad")
  C. Patients usually unaware of deficit
  D. Wernicke's area: temporal lobe (dominant hemisphere)
    1. Typically, strokes involving inferior division of the MCA
    2. Can be accompanied by contralateral homonymous superior quadrantanopia

IV. Other Aphasia
  A. Conduction: imparied repetition, preserved fluency and comprehension
  B. Global: impaired language production, comprehension, and repetition
  C. Anomic: impaired word-finding ability with preserved repetition, fluency, and comprehension
  D. Transcortical motor aphasia
    1. Resembles Broca's aphasia with preserved repetition
  E. Transcortical sensory aphasia
    1. Resembles Wernicke's aphasia with preserved repetition
  F. Transcortical mixed aphasia
    1. Impaired comprehension of spoken and written language
    2. Preserved repetition

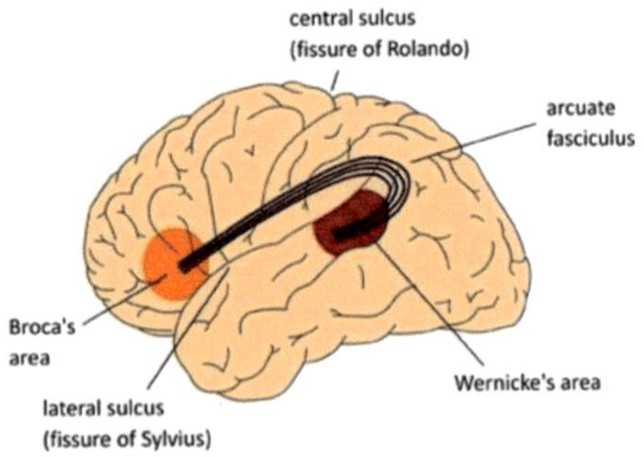

FIGURE 13.1.94 - Broca Area, Wernicke Area and Arcuate Fasciculus

V. Aphasia: Diagnosis
  A. Test patient's naming ability
  B. Patients will not be able to name objects
    1. E.g. being able to name a watch
  C. Ask patients to repeat a phrase ("no ifs ands or buts")
  D. Ask patients to read a phrase ("close your eyes") and do what it says
  E. Can ask patients to write a sentence

VI. Aphasia: Management
  A. Typically, regain most of their language abilities within first month
  B. Speech and language therapy
  C. Other measures are currently being studied
    1. Pharmacological therapy
    2. Transcranial electrical and magnetic stimulation

VII. Apraxia
  A. Inability to carry out a learned motor task despite ability to do so
    1. E.g. trying to hammer a nail, combing their hair
  B. Patient will struggle to mimic these actions
  C. Patients may use limbs as objects
    1. E.g. using entire hands as a comb

VIII. Agnosia
- A. Inability to recognize things despite having the sensory ability to do so
- B. May be able to describe specific features but not the object as a whole
- C. Visual agnosia: inability to recognize objects
    - 1. E.g. not recognizing a pen by looking at it
- D. Prosopagnosia: inability to recognize faces

IX. Neglect
- A. Lack of attention to one hemispace ("hemispatial neglect")
- B. Patients tend to be less aware of objects in one side of the world
- C. Typically involves non-dominant hemisphere of parietal lobe
- D. Patient may not be able to draw a clock correctly
- E. Most sensitive sign is extinction of double simultaneous stimulation
    - 1. Sensory stimuli are recognized one at a time but when both sides are stimulated only one side (non-neglected side) is felt

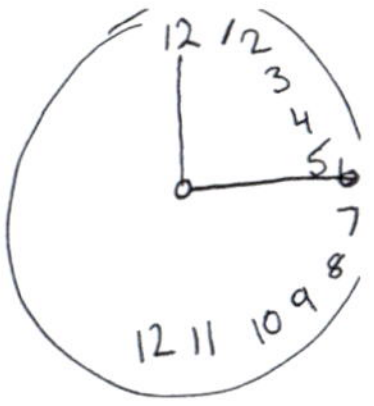

Dhru4you, Public domain, via Wikimedia Commons

FIGURE 13.1.95 - A Clock Drawn by a Person with Neglect

X. Gerstmann's Syndrome
- A. Constellation of issues with higher cortical function
    - 1. Agraphia, acalculia, finger agnosia, right-left confusion
- B. Involves inferior parietal lobe of dominant hemisphere (angular gyrus)

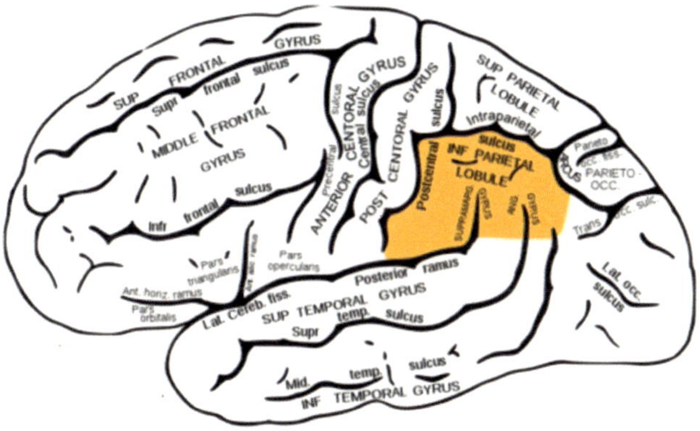

Gray, vectorized by Mysid, colourd by was_a_bee., Public domain, via Wikimedia Commons

FIGURE 13.1.96 - Area Affected in Gerstmann's Syndrome

Condition	Etiology/Location	Key Features
Broca's Aphasia	- Broca's area (frontal lobe), MCA stroke	- Impaired speech production
Wernicke's Aphasia	- Wernicke's area (temporal lobe), MCA stroke	- Impaired speech comprehension
Conduction Aphasia	- Arcuate fasciculus	- Impaired repetition - Preserved fluency and comprehension
Global Aphasia	- Large dominant hemispheric lesions affecting Broca's and Wernicke's areas	- Impaired repetition, fluency, comprehension
Anomic Aphasia	- Etiology unclear	- Impaired word-finding ability
Transcortical motor aphasia	- Supplementary motor area (frontal lobe); Broca's area intact	- Broca's aphasia but with preserved repetition
Transcortical sensory aphasia	- Inferior portion of left temporal lobe; Wernicke's area intact	- Wernicke's aphasia but with preserved repetition
Transcortical mixed aphasia	- Broca's area, Wernicke's area, arcuate fasciculus intact - Surrounding watershed areas affected	- Impaired comprehension of oral and written language - Preserved repetition
Gerstmann's Syndrome	- Inferior parietal lobe of dominant hemisphere; angular gyrus	- Agraphia, acalculia, finger agnosia, R-L confusion
Hemispatial neglect	- Inferior parietal lobe of non-dominant hemisphere	- Inability to recognize objects in one hemispace - Inability to draw a clock
Agnosia	- Sensory association area	- Impaired ability to recognize objects
Apraxia	- Frontal or parietal lobe of dominant hemisphere	- Impaired ability to perform learned motor task (e.g. hammering a nail, blowing out a candle, combing hair)

TABLE 13.1.12 - Aphasia, Neglect, Gerstmann's Syndrome, Agnosia, and Apraxia

REVIEW QUESTIONS

1. A 65-year-old woman is brought to her neurologist for follow-up examination. She is unable to follow instructions, repeat after the physician, or speak fluently without frequent word-finding difficulties. What type of aphasia does this patient most likely suffer from?

   - **This patient most likely has global aphasia.**
   - This woman lacks fluency, repetition, and comprehension.
   - This is consistent with the diagnosis of global aphasia.
   - It is important to note that if this patient was able to repeat after the physician, the likely diagnosis would change from global aphasia to transcortical mixed aphasia.
   - Hence, the key way to distinguish global aphasia from transcortical mixed aphasia is to assess the patient's ability to repeat.

2. Which three specific components of speech should be assessed in order to confidently distinguish between Broca, Wernicke, and conduction aphasia?

   - **In order to distinguish the three aphasia syndromes, it is important to assess the patient's fluency, repetition, and comprehension.**
   - If the patient has Broca aphasia, the patient will be able to comprehend; however, the patient will not be able to repeat or speak fluently.
   - If the patient has Wernicke aphasia, the patient will be able to speak fluently, however, the patient will not be able to repeat or comprehend a set of instructions.
   - If the patient has conduction aphasia, the patient will appear fluent and will be able to comprehend instructions, however, the patient will not be able to repeat.

3. A 64-year-old woman who works as an accountant comes to her primary care provider because of "brain fog" for the past 3 months. She says, "It's like I'm progressively forgetting how to do math!" She has a past medical history significant for hypertension, type 2 diabetes mellitus, and hyperlipidemia. Medications include lisinopril, metformin, and atorvastatin. Vital signs are all within normal limits. When the patient is asked to point to her right index finger, she points to her left ring finger. When the clinician looks through the review of systems charts that the patient was asked to fill out, he notices that it was left blank. This constellation of findings can most likely be attributed to a lesion in which of the following brain areas?

   A. Left frontal
   B. Left parietal
   C. Left temporal
   D. Right frontal
   E. Right parietal
   F. Right temporal

   - **The correct answer is option B.**
   - This patient is exhibiting the classic features of the Gerstmann's syndrome, which are acalculia, agraphia, finger agnosia, and inability to discriminate left from right.
   - Acalculia is suggested by her saying that she is progressively forgetting how to do math.
   - Agraphia is suggested by the fact that she did not fill out a review of systems charts.
   - Finger agnosia and inability to discriminate left from right are suggested by the fact that she was not able to point to her right index finger, instead pointing to her left ring finger.
   - Given all of these features, Gerstmann's syndrome is the most likely diagnosis. Gerstmann's syndrome occurs due to a problem in the inferior parietal lobe of the dominant hemisphere. In most people the dominant parietal lobe is the left parietal lobe.

Neurology | Section 21: Localizing Neurologic Lesions: Introduction

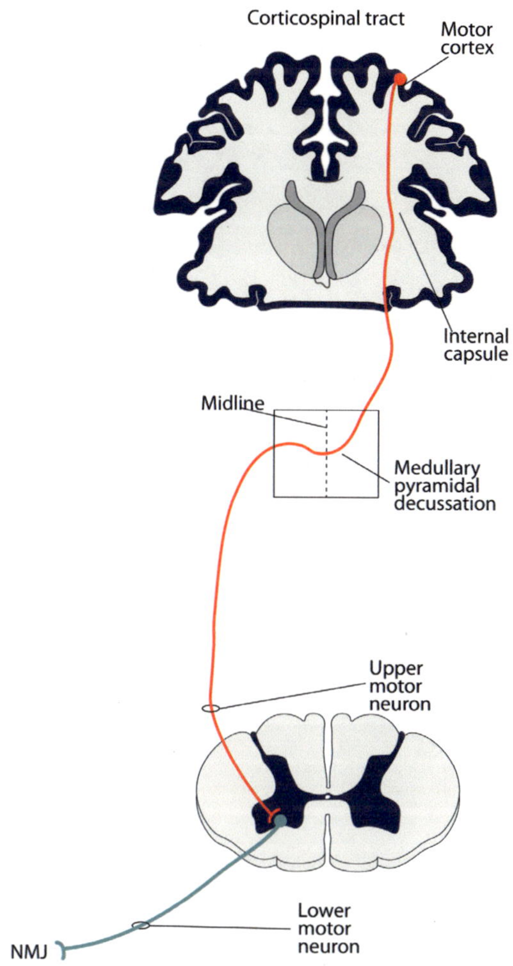

FIGURE 13.1.97 - The Corticospinal Tract

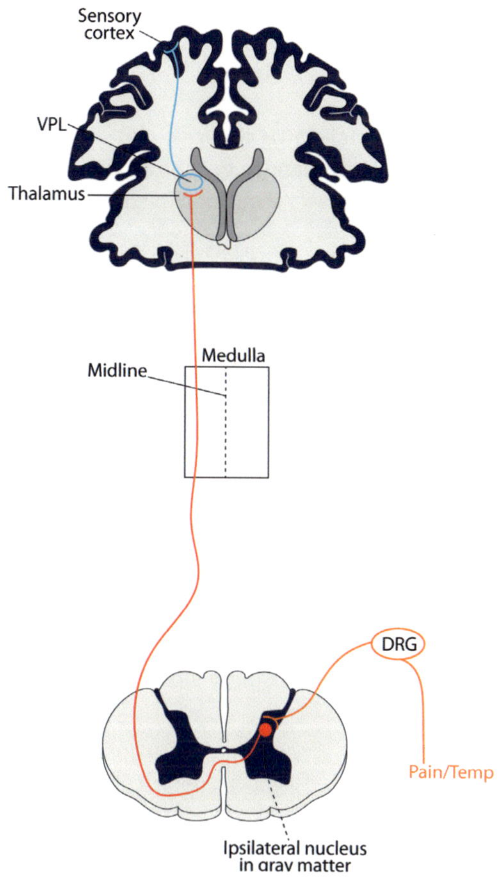

FIGURE 13.1.98 - Spinothalamic Tract

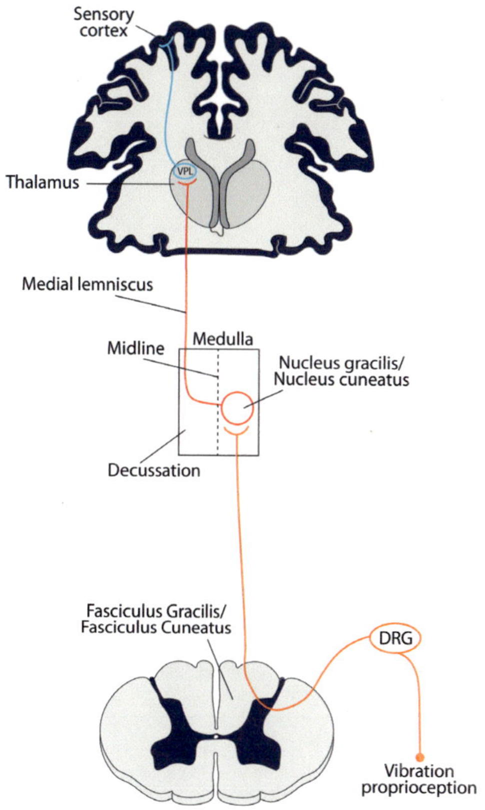

FIGURE 13.1.99 - Dorsal Column-Medial Lemniscus Pathway

I. Localizing Neurologic Lesions: Introduction
   A. UMN lesion (first-order neuron)
      1. Cerebral cortex
      2. Subcortex (e.g. internal capsule, thalamus)
      3. Brain stem
      4. Spinal cord
   B. Symptoms and signs of UMN lesion
      1. Spasticity
      2. Exaggerated DTRs (hyperreflexia)
      3. Babinski sign
   C. LMN lesion (second-order neuron)
      1. Anterior horn cells
      2. Peripheral neurons
   D. Symptoms and signs of LMN lesion
      1. Flaccid weakness
      2. Fasciculations
      3. Muscle atrophy
      4. Diminished/absent DTRs
   E. Ipsilateral vs. contralateral manifestations
   F. Lesion at or above the decussation → contralateral manifestations
   G. Lesion below the decussation → ipsilateral manifestations

Neurology | Section 22: Cerebral Cortex, Subcortex, Brainstem and Cerebellum

I. Cerebral Cortex Lesions
   A. Commonly caused by stroke (ischemic, hemorrhagic)
   B. Characteristic features
      1. Seizures
      2. Mental status changes
      3. Cortical signs (e.g. aphasia, agnosia, apraxia)
      4. Contralateral motor and somatosensory deficits

Condition	Key Features
MCA stroke	- Contralateral motor & somatosensory deficits in face & upper extremity - Aphasia (Broca's, Wernicke's, conduction) - Conjugate eye deviation toward lesion side - Contralateral homonymous hemianopia/quadrantanopia
ACA stroke	- Contralateral motor and somatosensory deficits in lower extremity - Urinary incontinence
Gerstmann syndrome (dominant parietal lobe)	- Agraphia, acalculia, finger agnosia, right-left disorientation
Lacunar stroke of thalamus (ventral posterior nuclei)	- Pure sensory stroke: contralateral sensory loss affecting face/arm/leg - Thalamic pain syndrome: paroxysmal burning pain, allodynia
Lacunar stroke of internal capsule (posterior limb)	- Pure motor hemiparesis: contralateral hemiparesis affecting face/arm/leg

TABLE 13.1.13 - Localization of Cortical and Subcortical Lesions

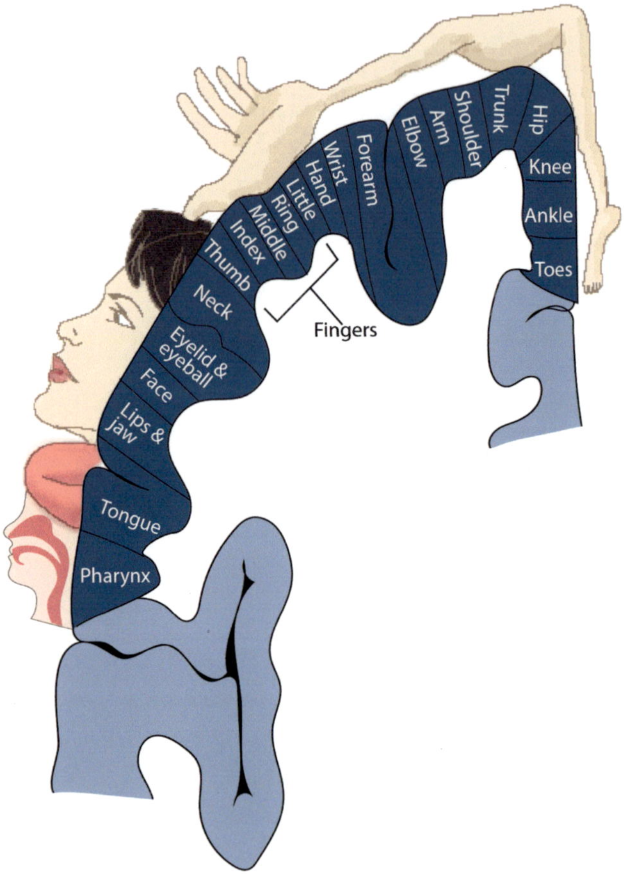

FIGURE 13.1.101 - The Homunculus

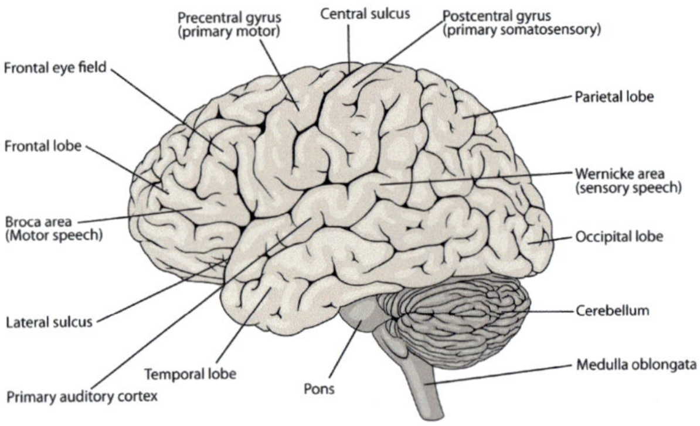

FIGURE 13.1.100 - Lateral Side of Cerebral Hemisphere

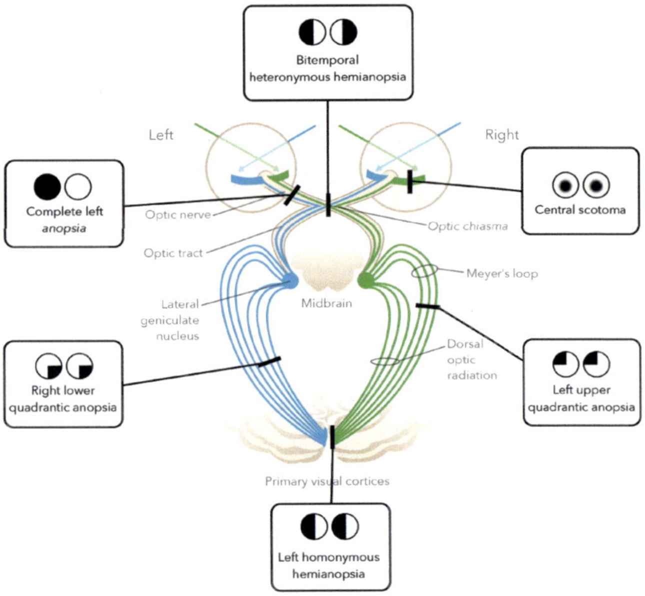

FIGURE 13.1.102 - The Optic Pathway

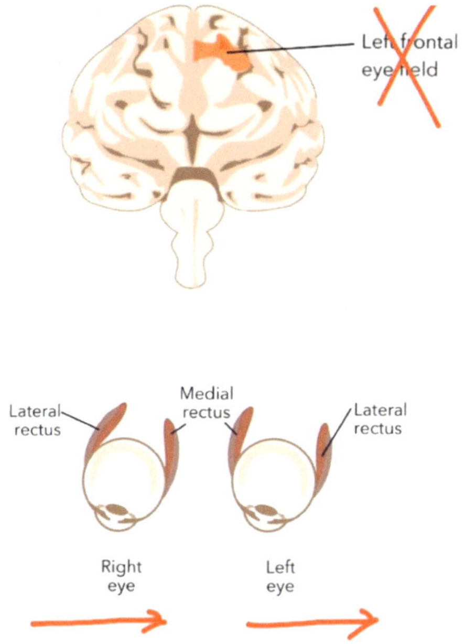

FIGURE 13.1.103 - Conjugate Eye Deviation Towards Lesion Side

II. Subcortical Lesions
   A. Lacunar stroke is an important cause
   B. Characteristic conditions
      1. Lesion affecting thalamus (VP nuclei): pure sensory stroke
      2. Lesion affecting internal capsule (posterior limb): pure motor hemiparesis
   C. No cortical signs, no cranial nerve deficits

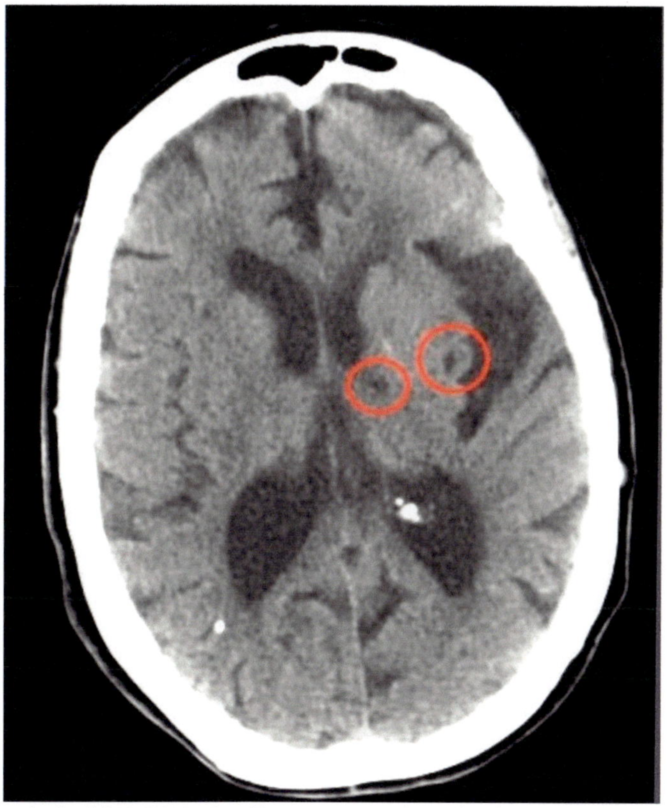

FIGURE 13.1.104- CT Scan of the Head: Lacunar Infarcts

III. Brainstem Lesions
   A. Etiology: ischemia, hemorrhage, trauma, neoplasms
   B. General features
      1. Contralateral hemiparesis affecting arm/leg
      2. Contralateral sensory loss affecting arm/leg
      3. Ipsilateral cranial nerve deficits

Condition	Key Features
Medial medullary syndrome	- Contralateral hemiparesis & loss of proprioception and vibratory sense (upper & lower extremities) - Ipsilateral bulbar features: tongue paralysis, tongue deviation toward lesion side
Lateral medullary syndrome (Wallenberg syndrome)	- Loss of pain & temperature sensation (contralateral arm/leg, ipsilateral face) - Ipsilateral bulbar features: dysphagia, dysarthria, hoarseness, ↓ gag reflex - Vertigo, ipsilateral limb ataxia - Ipsilateral Horner syndrome
Lateral pontine syndrome	- Loss of pain & temperature sensation (contralateral arm/leg, ipsilateral face) - Ipsilateral bulbar features: facial paralysis, ↓ lacrimation & salivation, ↓ taste from ⅔ anterior tongue - Vertigo, ipsilateral limb ataxia - Ipsilateral Horner syndrome

TABLE 13.1.14 - Localization of Brainstem Lesions

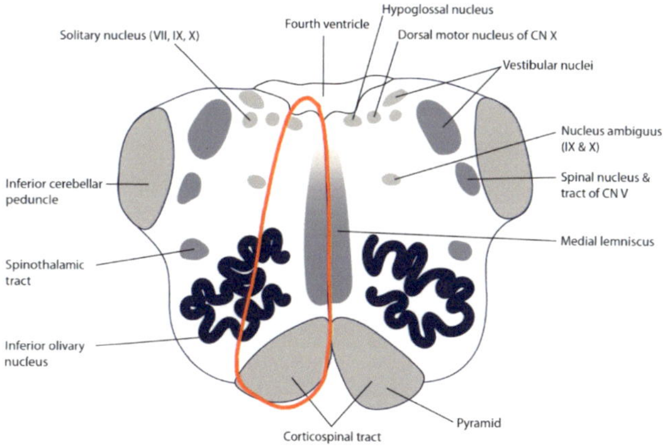

FIGURE 13.1.105 - Cross-Section of Medulla Oblongata: Area Affected in Medial Medullary Syndrome

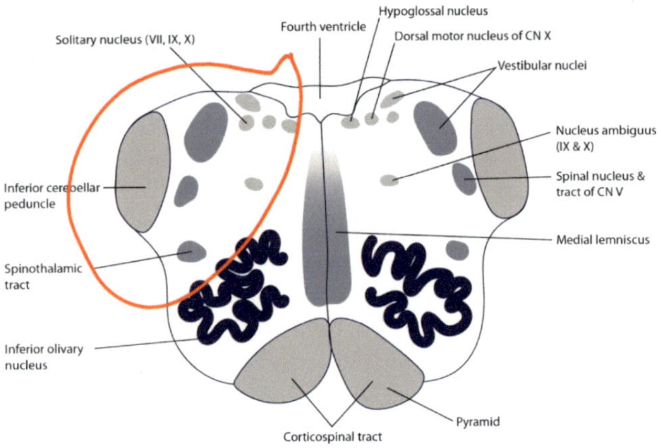

FIGURE 13.1.106 - Cross-Section of Medulla Oblongata: Area Affected in Lateral Medullary Syndrome

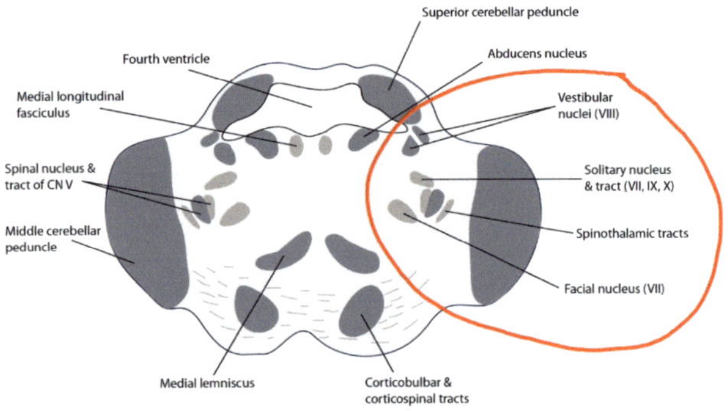

FIGURE 13.1.107 - Cross-Section of the Pons: Area Affected in Lateral Pontine Syndrome

IV. Cerebellar Lesions
   A. Etiology: ischemia, hemorrhage, neoplasms, alcohol intoxication
   B. Truncal/limb ataxia
   C. Staggering, wide-based gait
   D. Dysarthria, scanning speech
   E. Intention tremor
   F. Dysmetria, dysdiadochokinesia

REVIEW QUESTIONS

1. What is the difference between Broca's aphasia, Wernicke's aphasia, and conduction aphasia?
   - **Broca's aphasia is characterized by nonfluent speech, intact comprehension, and impaired repetition.**
   - Wernicke's aphasia is characterized by fluent speech, impaired comprehension, and impaired repetition.
   - Conduction aphasia, caused by damage to the arcuate fasciculus, is characterized by fluent speech, intact comprehension, and impaired repetition.
   - Broca's area is responsible for producing fluent speech and complete sentences.
   - Wernicke's area is responsible for comprehension of spoken language. The fluent speech of Wernicke's aphasia is typically of no sense, often referred to as "word salad".
   - Lastly, the arcuate fasciculus connects Wernicke's area to Broca's area.
   - All of these three structures should be intact for the repetition to be intact as well.

2. A 67-year-old woman is brought to the emergency department by her son because of a sudden onset of numbness 30 minutes ago. She has a long-standing history of uncontrolled hypertension. Physical examination shows loss of all types of sensation on the left half of her face and left side of her body. Muscle strength is 5/5 throughout the upper and lower extremities. Deep tendon reflexes are 2+ throughout. What is the most likely diagnosis?
   - **The most likely diagnosis is a pure sensory stroke due to lacunar infarct of thalamus.**
   - This patient presents with sudden loss of all types of sensation on the left half of the face and left side of the body.
   - She has a long-standing history of uncontrolled hypertension.
   - Muscle strength is 5/5 throughout the body, which is a normal finding. Deep tendon reflexes are 2+, which is also a normal finding.
   - Since this patient has only sensory symptoms, she likely experiences a pure sensory stroke, which is due to lacunar infarct of thalamus.

REVIEW QUESTIONS

3. A 72-year-old man is brought to the emergency department by his son due to sudden loss of balance 1 hour ago. He has a long-standing history of uncontrolled hypertension. Physical examination shows loss of pain and temperature sensation on the right side of the face and the left side of the body. Additionally, the patient has dysarthria and depressed gag reflex. Which is the most likely diagnosis in this patient?

   - **The most likely diagnosis is lateral medullary syndrome involving PICA.**
   - This elderly patient presents with the sudden loss of balance.
   - He has a long-standing history of hypertension.
   - There is loss of pain and temperature sensation on the right side of the face and the left side of the body. Additionally, the patient has dysarthria and depressed gag reflex.
   - All these signs and symptoms are consistent with the diagnosis of the lateral medullary syndrome, also known as Wallenberg syndrome, which is caused by decreased blood flow in the posterior inferior cerebellar artery (PICA).

4. An 82-year-old woman comes to urgent care because of tremor in her right hand that started 2 hours ago. Physical examination shows right-sided dysmetria on finger-to-nose test. Heel-to-shin test is abnormal when performed by the right leg. Rapid alternating movements of the right hand are also impaired. Which structure of the central nervous system is damaged in this patient?

   - **The cerebellum is damaged in this patient.**
   - This patient presents with an acute onset of tremor in her right hand.
   - Physical examination shows right-sided dysmetria on the finger-to-nose test. Heel-to-shin test is abnormal when performed by the right leg. Rapid alternating movements of the right hand are also impaired.
   - All of these are signs of cerebellar dysfunction.
   - As a general rule, the side of cerebellar dysfunction coincides with the side of presenting symptoms. Since the signs and symptoms are prominent on the right side, this patient likely has the right-sided cerebellar stroke.

5. A 75-year-old man is brought to the emergency department by his daughter because of sudden onset of weakness and urinary incontinence that started 2 hours ago. He was watching TV when he felt weakness in his right leg. He has a history of poorly controlled hypertension for the last 30 years. Physical examination shows 1/5 muscle strength and 5+ deep tendon reflexes in the right leg. Pain, temperature sensation, vibratory sensation, and proprioception are all diminished in the right leg. Which of the following vessels is most likely affected in this patient's condition?

   A. Right anterior cerebral artery
   B. Left anterior cerebral artery
   C. Right middle cerebral artery
   D. Left posterior cerebral artery

   - **The correct answer is option B.**
   - This patient presents with weakness in his right leg and urinary incontinence.
   - Physical exam shows 1/5 muscle weakness and 5+ deep tendon reflexes in the right leg. Such a severe weakness along with hyperreflexia indicate the upper motor neuron injury.
   - Pain, temperature sensation, vibratory sensation, and the proprioception are all diminished in the right leg (contralateral to side of the lesion).
   - Loss of all sensory modalities with UMN lesion and urinary incontinence likely indicate a cortical injury.
   - The primary motor and somatosensory cortices controlling the lower extremities fall in the vascular territory of the anterior cerebral artery. Since the pathways cross going up and down the brain, the right leg dysfunction is likely caused by damage to the left anterior cerebral artery.
   - Option A is incorrect because occlusion of the right anterior cerebral artery would present with left, rather than right leg dysfunction.
   - Option C is incorrect because occlusion of the right middle cerebral artery would present with motor weakness and the sensory disturbances of the left face and arm.
   - Option D is incorrect because occlusion of the left posterior cerebral artery would present with right homonymous hemianopia with macular sparing.

Neurology | Section 23: Spinal Cord, Peripheral Neurons, Neuromuscular Junction, Muscles, Diagnosis & Management

I. Localizing Lesions: Spinal Cord Lesions
   A. Etiology: infarction, trauma, infection, neoplasms
   B. Ipsilateral UMN-type motor deficit below the lesion level
   C. Ipsilateral LMN-type motor deficit at lesion level (anterior horn cell injury)
   D. Presence of sensory level: the lowest dermatome with intact pinprick and light touch sensation

Condition	Key Features
Anterior cord syndrome	- Bilateral hemiparesis at and below lesion level - Bilateral loss of pain and temperature sensation below the lesion level
Central cord syndrome	- Bilateral loss of pain and temperature sensation at lesion level - LMN-type motor deficits at lesion level
Brown-Sequard syndrome	- Ipsilateral hemiparesis at and below the lesion level - Contralateral loss of pain and temperature sensation below the lesion level - Ipsilateral loss of proprioception and vibratory sense at and below the lesion level - Ipsilateral Horner syndrome (cervical sympathetic pathway)

TABLE 13.1.15 - Classic Spinal Cord Lesions

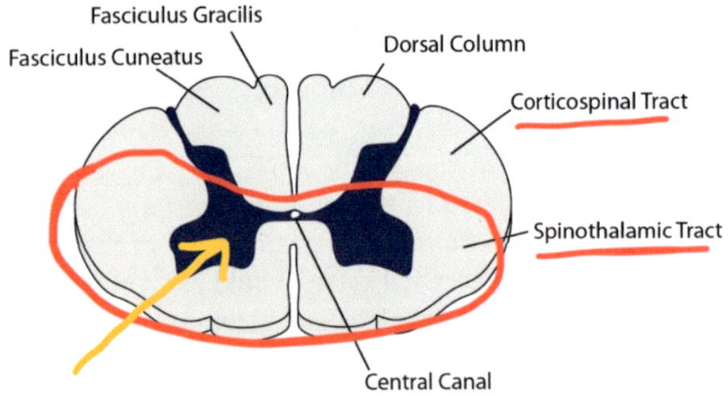

FIGURE 13.1.108 - Region Affected by Anterior Cord Syndrome

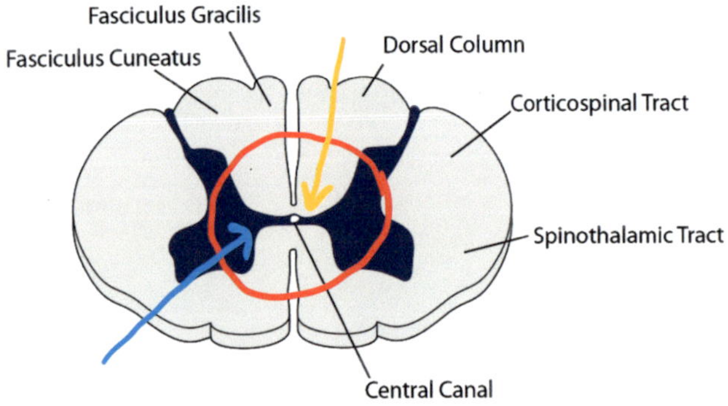

FIGURE 13.1.109 - Region Affected by Central Cord Syndrome

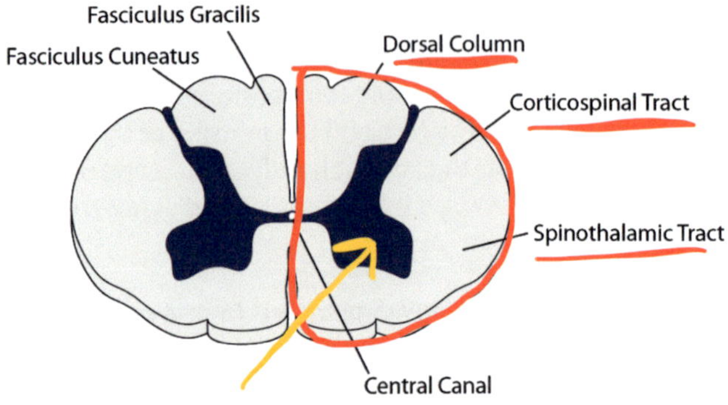

FIGURE 13.1.110 - Region Affected by Brown-Sequard Syndrome

II. Localizing Lesions: Peripheral Nerve Lesions
   A. Etiology: trauma, compression, diabetes mellitus, lead poisoning, chemotherapy (e.g. vincristine)
   B. Motor neuropathy
      1. Symptoms depends on affected myotome(s)
      2. LMN-type weakness, absent/diminished DTRs

III. Localizing Lesions: Peripheral Nerve Lesions
   A. Sensory neuropathy
      1. Symptoms depend on affected dermatome(s)
      2. Paresthesia, loss of pain and temperature sensation, impaired proprioception and vibratory sense

IV. Localizing Lesions: Neuromuscular Junction Lesions
   A. Etiology: myasthenia gravis, Lambert-Eaton myasthenic syndrome
   B. Muscle weakness
   C. Fatigability
   D. No muscle atrophy
   E. Sensation is intact

V. Localizing Lesions: Muscles Lesions (Myopathy)
   A. Etiology: duchenne muscular dystrophy, polymyositis, corticosteroids
   B. Symmetric muscle weakness, mainly proximal
   C. Sensation is intact
   D. Muscle atrophy and diminished DTRs in late disease

VI. Localizing Lesions: Diagnosis and Management
   A. Diagnosis
      1. Clinical examination is essential
      2. Imaging tests (e.g. MRI, CT)
      3. Nerve conduction and electromyographic (EMG) studies
   B. Management: treat the underlying cause

REVIEW QUESTIONS

1. A 59-year-old man comes to his primary care physician because of weakness for the last 2 weeks. Physical examination shows flaccidity in the upper extremity muscles and spasticity in the lower extremity muscles. The patient cannot feel pain and temperature below the lower neck. Proprioception and vibratory sensation are intact throughout the body. What is the most likely diagnosis?
   - **The most likely diagnosis is anterior cord syndrome.**
   - This patient has flaccidity in the upper extremity muscles and spasticity in the lower extremity muscles.
   - This pattern of weakness is consistent with the type of LMN deficit at the level of a spinal cord lesion and the type of UMN deficit below the level of the lesion, due to injury of anterior horn cells and corticospinal tracts respectively.
   - Additionally, the patient cannot feel the pain and temperature below the lower neck which indicates the damage of the spinothalamic tracts.
   - Proprioception and vibratory sensation are intact throughout the body which means that the dorsal columns of the spinal cord are spared.
   - Damage to all the tracts of the spinal cord except for the dorsal columns is consistent with the anterior cord syndrome.

2. How can myasthenia gravis and lambert-eaton myasthenic syndrome be differentiated from one another?
   - **Myasthenia gravis is caused by antibodies to the nicotinic acetylcholine receptors on the motor end plate and characterized by decremental muscle response on the electromyography and weakness of small muscles such as extraocular muscles.**
   - **Lambert-Eaton myasthenic syndrome is caused by antibodies to the presynaptic calcium channels and characterized by incremental muscle response on the electromyography and weakness of large muscles such as shoulder muscles. Lambert-Eaton myasthenic syndrome is also characterized by autonomic symptoms like dry mouth and erectile dysfunction.**
   - Decremental muscle response on the electromyography means that muscle contraction weakens after every single nerve depolarization.
   - This is because successive nerve depolarizations deplete acetylcholine in the presynaptic terminals.
   - Therefore, low levels of acetylcholine can no longer displace the antibodies on the motor end plate.
   - Incremental muscle response on the electromyography means that muscle contraction strengthens after every single nerve depolarization.
   - This is because successive nerve depolarizations cause accumulation of sufficient calcium in the presynaptic terminals.
   - Therefore, presynaptic terminals start releasing acetylcholine and the muscle contraction strengthens.
   - Myasthenia gravis is characterized by weakness of small muscles because small muscles contract very frequently so acetylcholine quickly gets depleted in the corresponding nerves.
   - Lambert-Eaton myasthenic syndrome is characterized by weakness of large muscles because large muscles do not contract frequently so it takes time for the corresponding nerves to reach sufficient intracellular calcium levels in order to release acetylcholine.
   - Lambert-Eaton myasthenic syndrome is also characterized by autonomic symptoms like dry mouth and erectile dysfunction because the inability to release acetylcholine from the presynaptic terminals also affects the parasympathetic nerve fibers.

REVIEW QUESTIONS

3. A 38-year-old woman is brought to the emergency department via ambulance because of severe burns on both hands which occurred 30-minutes ago. She is a chef, and she burned her hands by accidentally spilling hot oil. She did not feel any pain but called the ambulance due to severe swelling and redness. Past medical history is significant for a motor vehicle accident 3 months ago. Physical examination shows second degree burns on the dorsal surfaces of her hands. Pain and temperature sensation is diminished in both upper extremities but is intact in the lower extremities. Physical examination also shows upper extremity weakness and 1+ biceps reflexes bilaterally. Knee and ankle reflexes are normal. Which of the following is the most likely diagnosis?

   A. Anterior cord syndrome
   B. Brown-Sequard syndrome
   C. Central cord syndrome
   D. Amyotrophic lateral sclerosis

- **The correct answer is option C.**
- This patient did not feel any pain while accidentally spilling the hot oil on her hands.
- Pain and temperature sensation is diminished in both upper extremities but is intact in the lower extremities.
- Upper extremity reflexes are diminished evidenced by 1+ biceps reflexes.
- However, the knee and ankle reflexes are normal.
- Bilateral loss of pain and temperature sensation along with the lower motor neuron signs at the level of the lesion is consistent with central cord syndrome.
- The central cord syndrome likely developed as a result of spinal trauma after the motor vehicle accident 3 months ago.
- Option A is incorrect because the anterior cord syndrome is characterized by bilateral loss of pain and temperature sensation, bilateral lower motor neuron weakness at the level of the lesion, and the bilateral upper motor neuron weakness below the level of the lesion.
- Option B is incorrect because Brown-Sequard syndrome is characterized by contralateral loss of pain and temperature sensation, ipsilateral lower motor neuron weakness at the level of the lesion, and an ipsilateral upper motor neuron weakness below the level of the lesion.
- Option D is incorrect because amyotrophic lateral sclerosis is characterized by bilateral lower motor neuron weakness at the level of the cord demyelination, and the bilateral upper motor neuron weakness below the level of the demyelination. However, all sensations are normal in amyotrophic lateral sclerosis.

Neurology | Section 24: Intracranial Hemorrhage: Subdural & Epidural Hematoma

I. Subdural Hematoma: Definition
   A. Collection of blood between dura mater and arachnoid mater
   B. May be acute or chronic

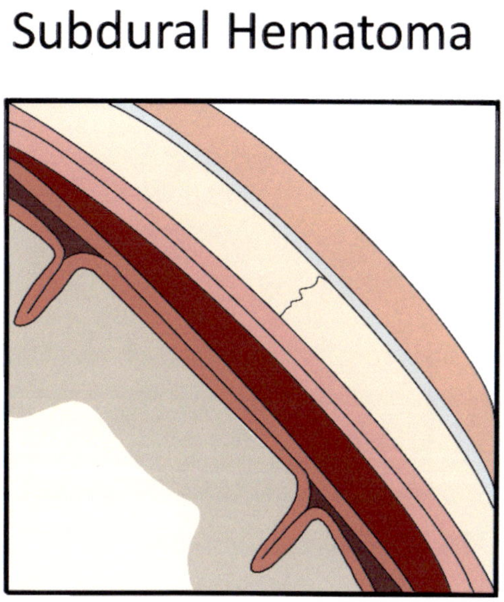

FIGURE 13.1.111 - Subdural Hematoma

II. Subdural Hematoma: Etiology
   A. Head trauma (most common cause)
   B. Anticoagulation
   C. Cerebral atrophy
   D. Child abuse (shaken baby syndrome)

III. Subdural Hematoma: Pathophysiology
   A. Tearing of bridging veins in subdural space → extravasation of blood at a relatively slow rate
   B. Bleeding may cross cranial suture lines but not the midline

IV. Subdural Hematoma: Clinical Presentation
   A. A history of trauma several days or weeks before
   B. Lethargy and confusion
   C. Impaired consciousness
   D. Focal neurologic deficits (e.g. hemiparesis)

V. Subdural Hematoma: Diagnosis
   A. Non-contrast CT of the head
      1. Crescent-shaped lesion that can cross suture lines
      2. Acute bleeding: hyperdense (light)
      3. Chronic bleeding: hypodense (dark)

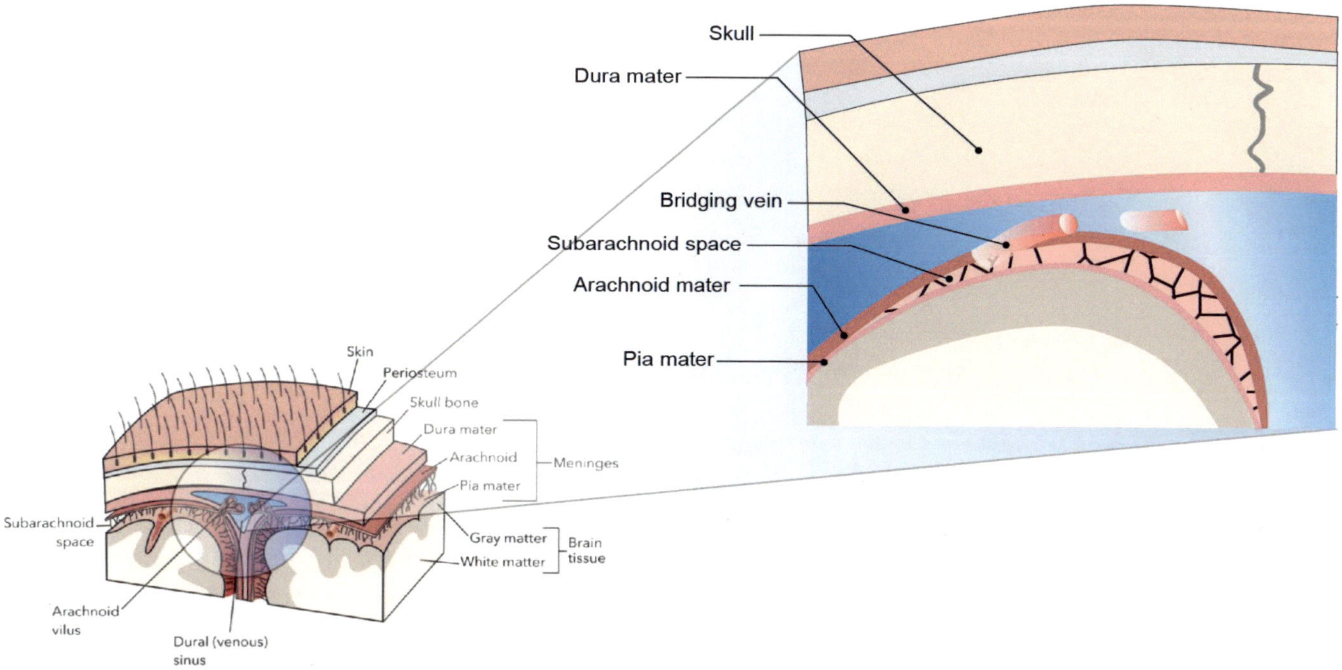

FIGURE 13.1.112 - Bridging Veins

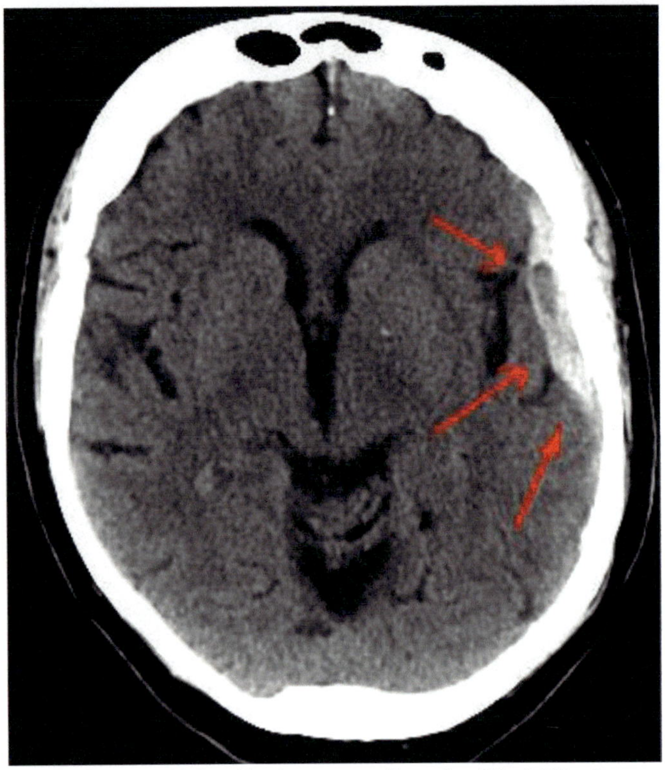

FIGURE 13.1.113 - CT Scan of the Head: Acute Subdural Hematoma

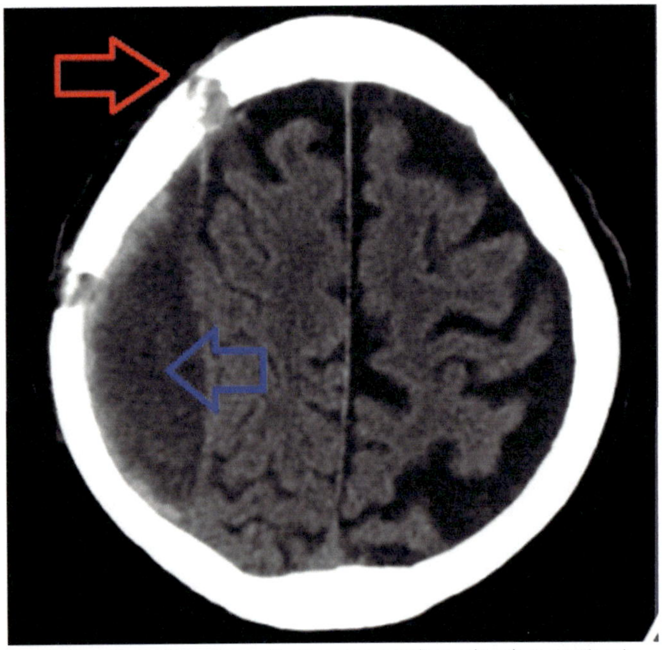

FIGURE13.1.114 - CT Scan of the Head: Chronic Subdural Hematoma

B. Subdural Hematoma: Management
   1. Subdural hematomas can regress spontaneously
   2. Hematoma evacuation if severe
   3. Large hematoma (i.e. 10 mm or greater)
   4. Brain herniation (i.e. > 5 mm midline shift)
   5. Neurological deterioration
   6. Failure of conservative management

VI. Epidural Hematoma: Definition
   A. Collection of blood between the dura mater and the periosteum

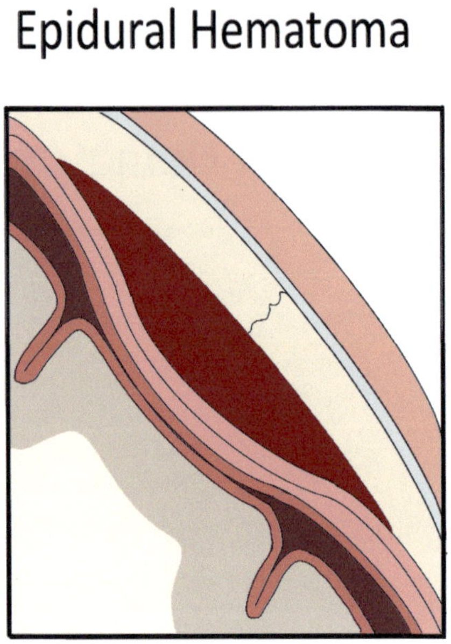

FIGURE 13.1.115 - Epidural Hematoma

VII. Epidural Hematoma: Etiology
   A. Most commonly caused by severe, acute head trauma (e.g. motor vehicle accidents)
   B. Occasionally caused by non-traumatic conditions
      1. Coagulopathies
      2. Malignancies
      3. Vascular malformation

VIII. Epidural Hematoma: Pathophysiology
   A. Severe head trauma, especially to the pterion → tearing of the middle meningeal artery → bleeding into the epidural space

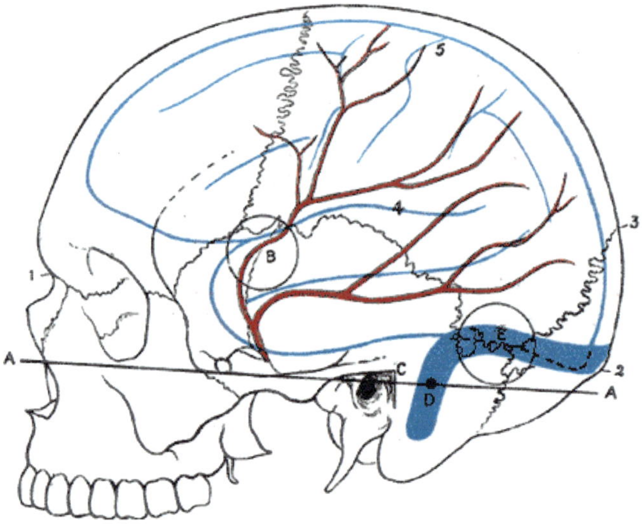

FIGURE 13.1.116 - Pterion and Middle Meningeal Artery

IX. Epidural Hematoma: Clinical Presentation
   A. History of trauma minutes to hours prior to presentation
   B. A lucid interval is common
      1. Brief loss of consciousnesses after trauma → lucid interval → deterioration of neurologic function
   C. Bleeding leads to high intracranial pressure and possible brain herniation (e.g. ipsilateral dilated pupil, contralateral hemiparesis)

X. Epidural Hematoma: Diagnosis
   A. Non-contrast CT of the head
      1. Lens-shaped (biconvex) hyperdensity
      2. Does not cross suture lines
      3. Skull fracture may be present

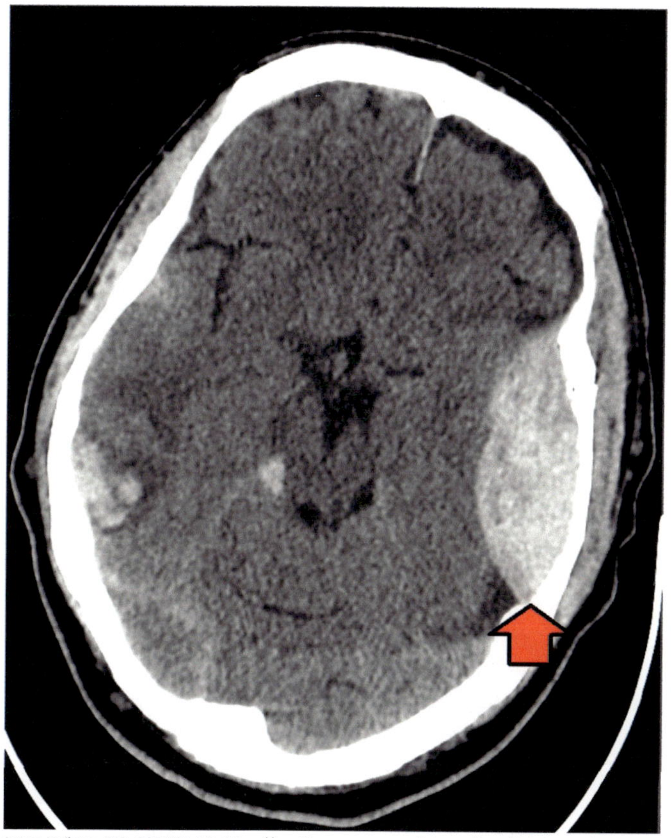

FIGURE 13.1.117 - CT Scan of the Head: Epidural Hematoma

XI. Epidural Hematoma: Management
   A. Emergent burrhole craniotomy with ligation of the bleeding artery
      1. Relieves high intracranial pressure and prevents herniation

REVIEW QUESTIONS ?

1. A 70-year-old woman is brought to the physician by her daughter due to excessive sleepiness for the past month. She has a medical history of chronic alcoholism and frequent falls due to alcohol intoxication. Her serum TSH level is normal and depression screening questionnaire is unremarkable. Physical examination shows right hemiparesis which was absent on the last check-up. What is the next best step in the diagnosis of this patient?
   - **The next best step is a non-contrast CT scan of the head.**
   - This elderly woman presents with excessive sleepiness for the past month.
   - She has a past medical history of chronic alcoholism and frequent falls due to alcohol intoxication.
   - Physical examination shows right hemiparesis which was absent on the last check-up.
   - Her serum TSH level is normal, and depression screening questionnaire is unremarkable, which makes underlying hypothyroidism and depression unlikely.
   - Sleepiness and the new-onset focal neurological deficits in a patient with frequent falls raises suspicion for subdural hematoma.
   - The best next step in the diagnosis of the patient with suspected subdural hematoma is non-contrast head CT scan.

2. A 17-year-old man is brought to the emergency department via ambulance and is unresponsive after being involved in an altercation that occurred 1 hour ago. Friends report that he was hit on the left side of his head by a baseball bat. After initial loss of consciousness, the patient recovered for several minutes. However, he lost consciousness again in the ambulance. Physical examination shows a dilated left pupil. What findings are expected on a non-contrast head CT scan of this patient?

REVIEW QUESTIONS

- **A non-contrast head CT scan in the patient with epidural hematoma typically shows the lens-shaped hyperdensity that does not cross the suture lines.**
- This young man is brought unresponsive after being involved in an altercation.
- He was hit on the left side of his head by a baseball bat.
- After initial loss of consciousness, the patient recovered for several minutes. However, he lost consciousness again in the ambulance. This phenomenon is known as lucid interval.
- Physical examination shows dilated left pupil indicating the imminent risk of brain herniation.
- The lucid interval and focal neurological deficits after head trauma raise a strong suspicion for epidural hematoma.

3. A 77-year-old female is brought to the emergency department by her daughter due to recent onset of lethargy and confusion. While performing a physical exam the patient appears to be slipping in and out of consciousness. Her daughter is with her and mentions a minor fall about a week ago, but the patient had seemed fine until now. A non-contrast head CT is ordered to get a closer look at what is going on with the patient. Results show a crescent-shaped lesion that does cross suture lines but not the midline. What is the pathophysiology behind this patient's current presentation?

   A. Tearing of bridging veins
   B. Severe head trauma
   C. Ruptured aneurysm
   D. Hypertension

- **The correct answer is option A.**
- This elderly woman has lethargy, confusion, and loss of consciousness.
- She had a minor fall one week ago.
- Non-contrast head CT shows a crescent-shaped lesion which crosses suture lines but not the midline.
- Based on the patient's head CT, she has a subdural hematoma which is often caused by tearing of the bridging veins during a minor fall in a patient with cerebral atrophy such as an elderly patient.
- Option B is incorrect because severe head trauma is the typical cause of an epidural hematoma which looks lens-shaped on CT scan and does not cross suture lines.
- Option C is incorrect because a ruptured aneurysm is the typical cause of a subarachnoid hemorrhage which often presents as an acute onset of the worst headache of a patient's life.
- Option D is incorrect because hypertension is the typical cause of an intraparenchymal hemorrhage which often results in ischemia to the basal ganglia.

Neurology | Section 25: Intracranial Hemorrhage: Subarachnoid & Intraparenchymal Hemorrhage

I. Subarachnoid Hemorrhage: Definition
   A. Bleeding into the subarachnoid space
      1. Between the pia mater and the arachnoid mater
      2. The space that houses most cerebrospinal fluid

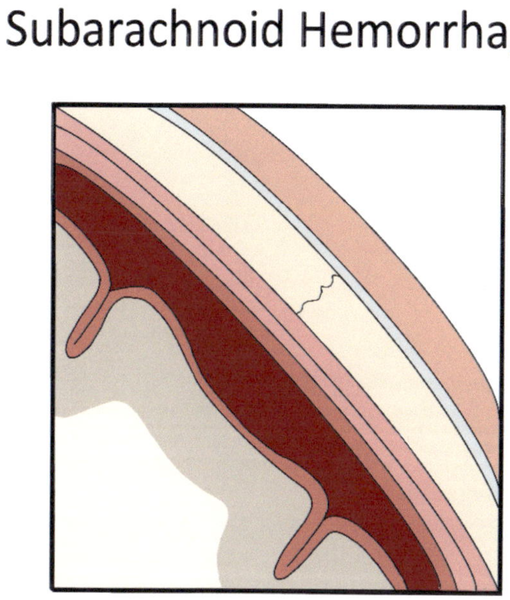

FIGURE 13.1.118 - Subarachnoid Hemorrhage

II. Subarachnoid Hemorrhage: Etiology
   A. Ruptured intracranial aneurysm (most commonly berry aneurysm)
      1. Usually spontaneous
   B. Arteriovenous malformation

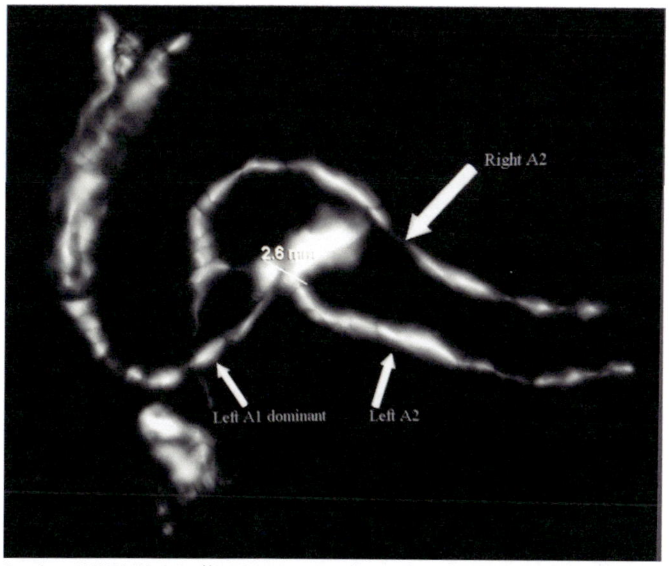

FIGURE 13.1.119 - CT Angiography: Berry Aneurysm

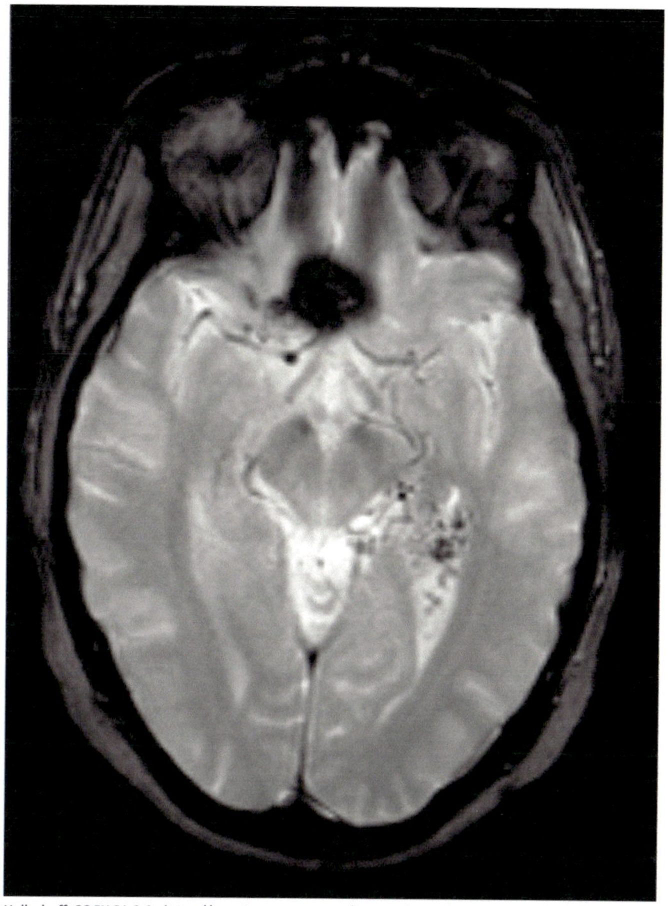

FIGURE 13.1.120 - MRI of the Brain: AV Malformation

III. Subarachnoid Hemorrhage: Risk Factors
   A. Smoking
   B. Hypertension
   C. Substance use (e.g. cocaine and methamphetamine)

IV. Subarachnoid Hemorrhage: Clinical Presentation
   A. Severe, sudden headache that doesn't respond to NSAIDs
      1. "The worst headache of my life"
   B. Meningitis-like signs (e.g. neck stiffness, photophobia)
   C. Cranial nerve deficits: enlarging or ruptured aneurysm compressing a nerve (e.g. CN III and CN II palsies)

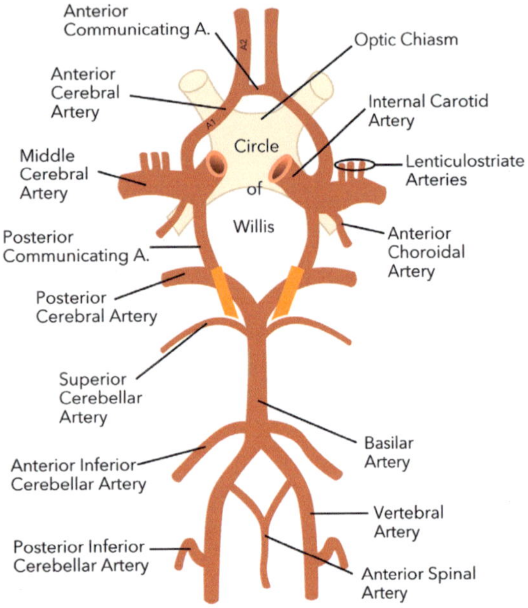

FIGURE 13.1.121 - Circle of Willis

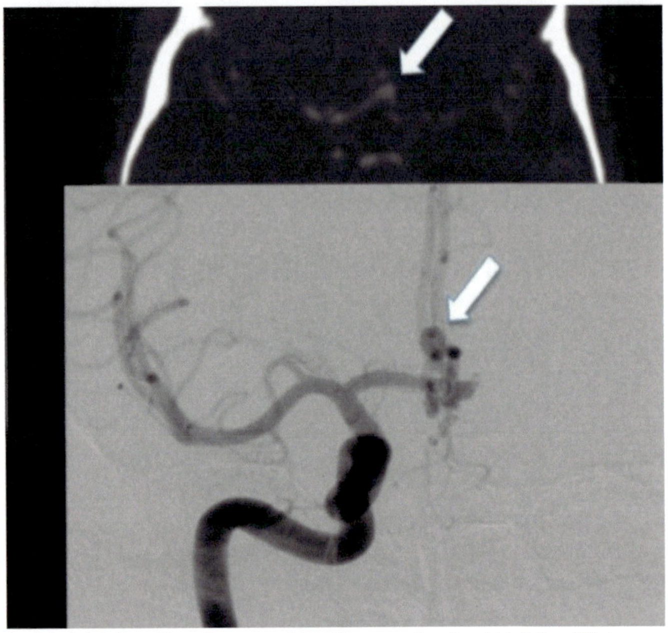

FIGURE 13.1.123 - CTA: Subarachnoid Hemorrhage and Arterial Aneurysm

V. Subarachnoid Hemorrhage: Diagnosis
   A. The best initial test is a non-contrast head CT
      1. Hyperintensity in the subarachnoid space
      2. If head CT is positive, perform angiography
   B. Lumbar puncture
      1. Very sensitive for subarachnoid hemorrhage
      2. Performed if CT is negative but there is a strong suspicion
      3. CSF findings: xanthochromia, elevated RBC count

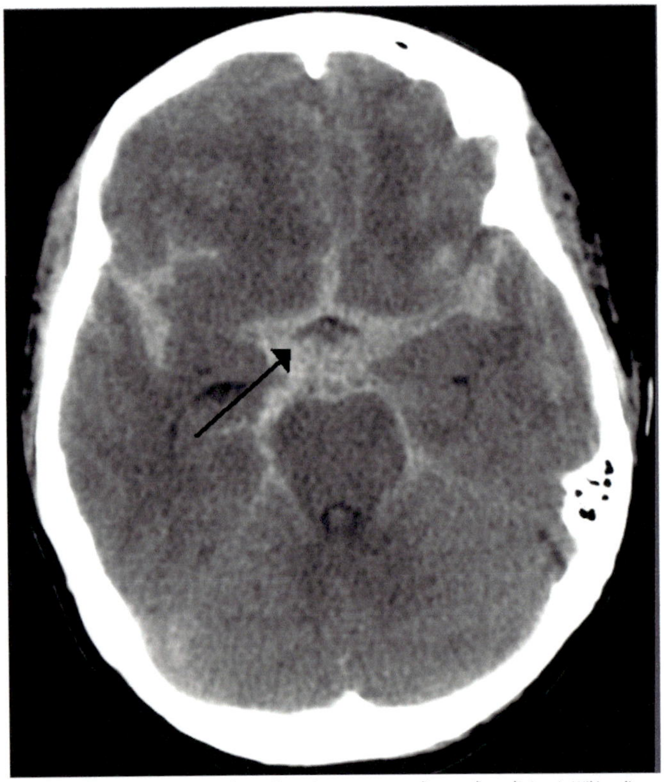

FIGURE 13.1.122 - CT Scan of the Head: Subarachnoid Hemorrhage

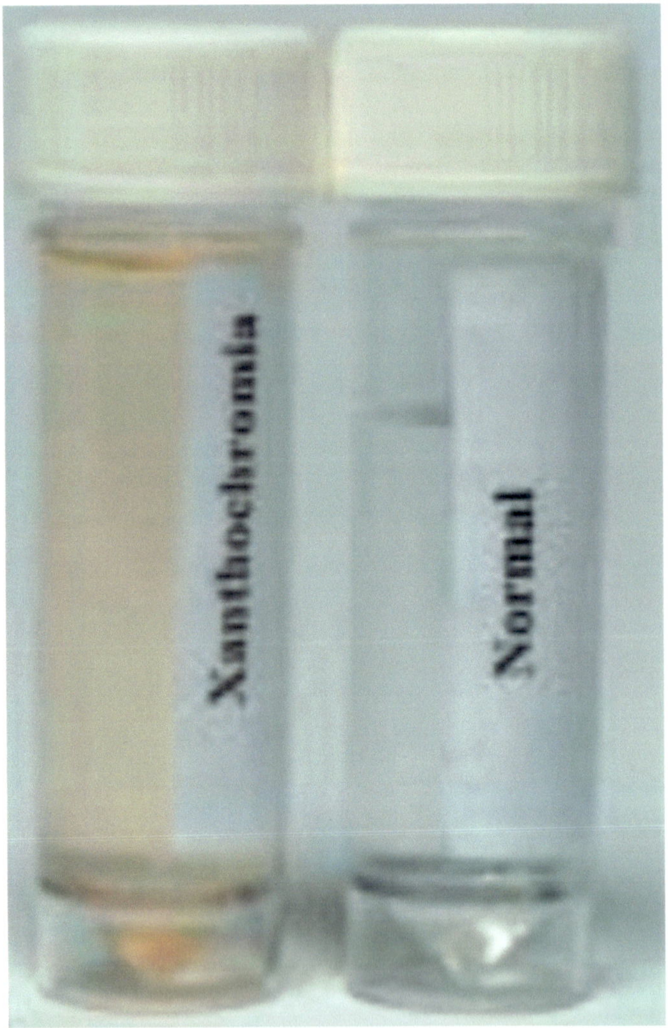

FIGURE 13.1.124 - Xanthochromia

VI. Subarachnoid Hemorrhage: Management
  A. Supportive therapy (e.g. airway management, breathing, IV fluids)
  B. Anticoagulation reversal, blood pressure control
  C. Emergent surgery: endovascular coiling, microsurgical clipping
  D. Cerebral vasospasm may occur several days later
    1. Vasospasm leads to ischemia
    2. Prevent with nimodipine

VII. Intraparenchymal Hemorrhage: Definition
  A. Also known as intracerebral hemorrhage
  B. Bleeding within the parenchyma due to rupture of blood vessels in the brain

Intraparenchymal Hemorrhage

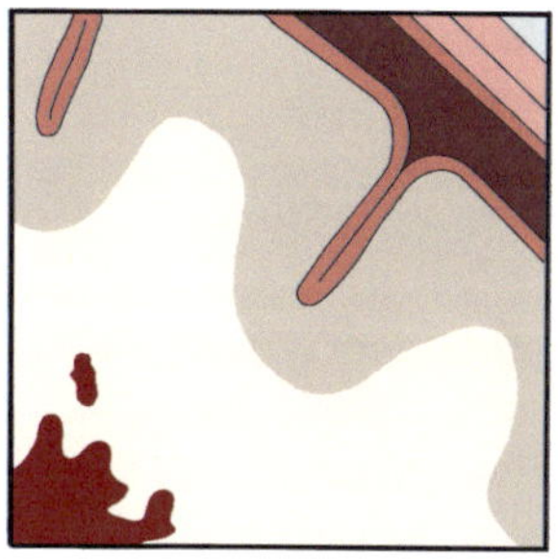

FIGURE 13.1.125 - Intraparenchymal Hemorrhage

VIII. Intraparenchymal Hemorrhage: Etiology
  A. Hypertension (most common cause of spontaneous hemorrhage)
  B. Cerebral amyloid angiopathy (most common in elderly)
  C. Arteriovenous malformations (most common in children)
  D. Coagulopathies (e.g. anticoagulation medications, hemophilia)
  E. HSV encephalitis
  F. Tumors, drugs (e.g. cocaine, methamphetamine)
  G. Head trauma

IX. Intraparenchymal Hemorrhage: Pathophysiology
  A. Chronic hypertension → hypertrophy of the tunica media and formation of lipofibrous deposits (i.e. lipohyalinosis) in the walls of lenticulostriate arteries → formation of Charcot-Bouchard aneurysms which eventually rupture → lacunar strokes affecting the basal ganglia (e.g. putamen, thalamus)
  B. Cerebral amyloid angiopathy
    1. Amyloid deposition in the walls of blood vessels in the brain → vessels are weakened and prone to bleeding → hemorrhage within one of the cerebral hemispheres (i.e. spontaneous lobar hemorrhage)
  C. Arteriovenous malformation
    1. Abnormal connections between arteries and veins (arteries anastomose with veins without capillary beds) → high-pressure system → aneurysms and spontaneous bleeding

X. Intraparenchymal Hemorrhage: Clinical Presentation
  A. Symptoms progress over minutes to hours
  B. Neurologic deficits worsen over time due to the expanding hematoma
    1. The deficit depends on the part of the brain that is affected
  C. High intracranial pressure is a late finding (e.g. nausea, bradycardia, impaired consciousness)
  D. If the hemorrhage affects the putamen:
    1. Contralateral hemiparesis
    2. Eyes deviated to the side of the hematoma
  E. If the hemorrhage affects the thalamus:
    1. Contralateral hemisensory loss
    2. Eyes deviated to the opposite side of the hematoma

XI. Intraparenchymal Hemorrhage: Diagnosis
  A. Non-contrast head CT
    1. Hyperdense area within the brain parenchyma
    2. Hypodense if it is chronic

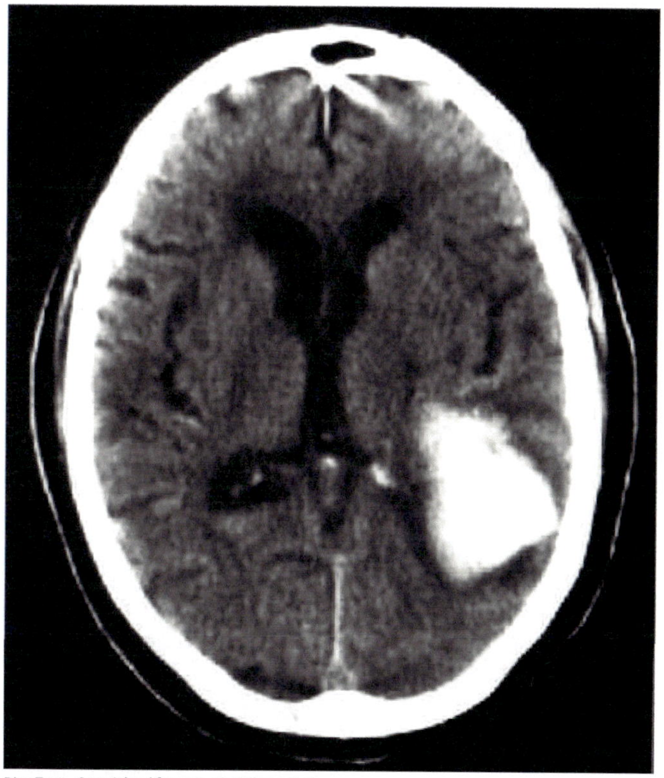

Diag Team, Copyrighted free use, via Wikimedia Commons

FIGURE 13.1.126 - CT Scan of the Head: Intracerebral Hemorrhage

XII. Intraparenchymal Hemorrhage: Management
  A. Most cases are managed conservatively
    1. Airway maintenance
    2. Cardiovascular support
    3. Anticoagulation reversal
    4. Blood pressure control
  B. Surgical hematoma evacuation +/- decompressive craniotomy (e.g. signs of brain herniation, deteriorating neurologic deficits)

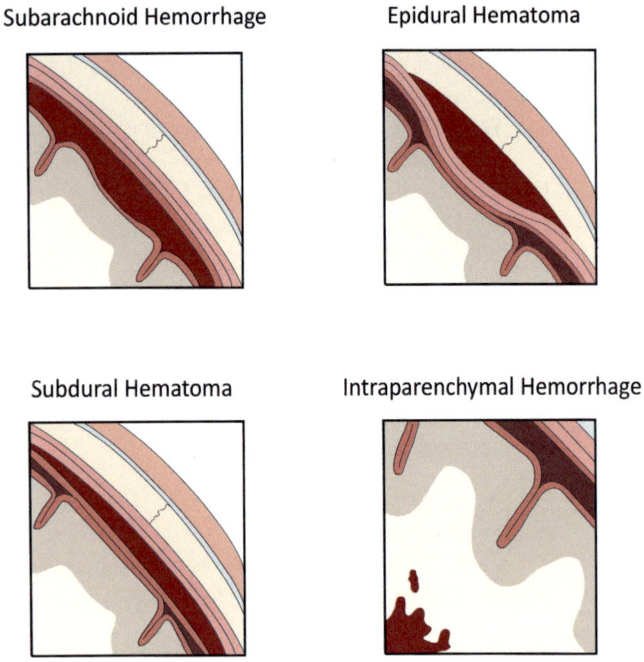

FIGURE 13.1.127 - Intracranial Hemorrhage

REVIEW QUESTIONS

1. A 35-year-old woman is brought to the emergency department by her partner because of a severe headache for the past 2 hours. The headache started suddenly while the patient was cooking. Physical examination shows neck rigidity and positive Kernig sign. Vital signs are unremarkable. A non-contrast head CT scan is obtained and unrevealing. What is the next best step in management of this patient?

- **The next best step in management is to perform a lumbar puncture.**
- This young woman presents with a sudden-onset severe headache for the past 2 hours.
- Physical examination shows neck rigidity and positive Kernig sign suggesting meningeal irritation.
- However, the patient is afebrile making meningitis unlikely.
- Sudden-onset severe headache along with meningeal irritation raises strong suspicion for a subarachnoid hemorrhage.
- The non-contrast head CT scan is unremarkable.
- If the clinical suspicion for subarachnoid hemorrhage is still high after unremarkable non-contrast head CT scan, a lumbar puncture should be performed.
- Lumbar puncture in the case of subarachnoid hemorrhage usually shows increased red blood cell count due to hemorrhage and xanthochromia due to hemoglobin breakdown into bilirubin.

REVIEW QUESTIONS

2. A 65-year-old man is brought to the emergency department by his daughter because of a severe headache for the past 4 hours. He has a past medical history of chronic alcoholism and uncontrolled hypertension. Vital signs include temperature of 98.6° F (37° C), blood pressure of 190/130 mmHg, heart rate of 89 beats/min, and respiratory rate of 14 breaths/min. Physical examination shows right-sided hemiparesis and left-sided deviation of both eyes. Non-contrast head CT scan shows expanding hyperdense mass in the left-sided brain parenchyma. Which of the following structures is most likely affected in this patient?

   A. Thalamus
   B. Putamen
   C. Cerebellum
   D. Septum pellucidum

- **The correct answer is option B.**
- This man with chronic alcoholism and uncontrolled hypertension presents with a severe headache for the past 4 hours.
- His vital signs are significant for hypertension of 190/130 mmHg. The blood pressure more than 180/120 mmHg along with signs of end-organ damage, like in this patient, is called the hypertensive emergency.
- Physical exam shows right-sided hemiparesis and left-sided deviation of both eyes.
- Non-contrast head CT scan shows expanding hyperdense mass in the left-sided brain parenchyma.
- All of these findings suggest the diagnosis of intraparenchymal hemorrhage due to malignant hypertension.
- The most likely site of intraparenchymal hemorrhage in this patient is the putamen. This is because putaminal hemorrhage is associated with contralateral hemiparesis and ipsilateral deviation of both eyes.
- Option A is incorrect because thalamic hemorrhage is associated with contralateral hemisensory loss and contralateral deviation of both eyes.
- Option C is incorrect because cerebellar hemorrhage is associated with cerebellar signs like ataxia, dysdiadochokinesia, and dysmetria which are absent in this patient.
- Option D is incorrect because septum pellucidum is an ultra-thin membrane separating the lateral ventricles from each other. It is typically not involved in the intraparenchymal hemorrhage.

I. Migraine: Definition
   A. Episodic severe primary headache disorder
   B. Mostly occurs in females
   C. May have a hereditary pattern

II. Migraine: Pathophysiology
   A. Abnormal activation of trigeminovascular system → increase in release of vasoactive mediators and neuropeptides (e.g. CGRP) → neurogenic inflammation and vasodilation → migraine headache

III. Migraine: Clinical Features
   A. Prodrome phase
      1. 24-48 hours prior to headache onset
      2. Examples include depression, irritation, food cravings
   B. Aura
      1. Focal neurologic symptoms typically preceding the headache
      2. Most commonly visual (e.g. flashes of light, scotoma)
      3. Can be auditory, somatosensory, or motor
   C. Migraine headache
      1. Throbbing, pulsating
      2. Mostly unilateral, can be bilateral in children
      3. Duration: 4 to 72 hours
      4. Photophobia, phonophobia, nausea, vomiting
      5. May be relieved by darkness and silence
   D. Postdrome phase (e.g. feelings of exhaustion)
   E. Migraine attacks can be triggered by emotional stress, menstruation, weather changes, lack of food or sleep

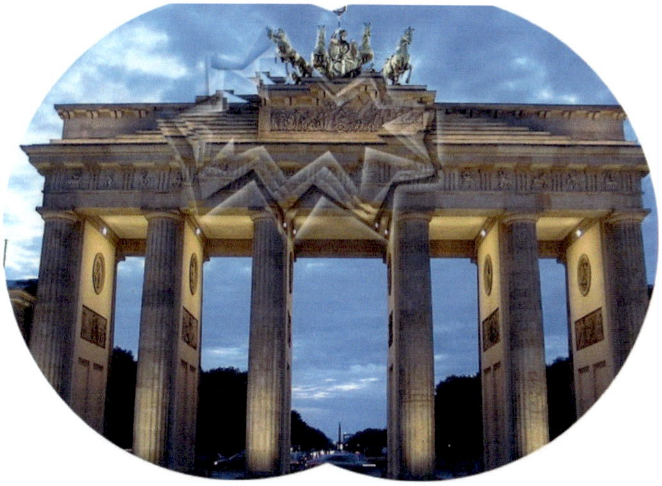

FIGURE 13.1.128 - Visual Aura

IV. Migraine: Diagnosis
   A. Mainly dependent on history and clinical presentation
   B. Imaging to rule out other causes (e.g. brain lesions, pseudotumor cerebri)

V. Migraine: Management
   A. Abortive therapy
      1. NSAIDs (e.g. aspirin, ketorolac), acetaminophen
      2. Triptans (e.g. sumatriptan)
         a) 5-HT1B/1D receptor agonists
      3. Ergots (e.g. ergotamine, parenteral dihydroergotamine)
         a) 5-HT1B/1D receptor agonists, alpha-adrenergic blocker
      4. Simultaneous use of triptans and ergots is contraindicated (risk of serotonin syndrome and coronary vasospasm)
      5. CGRP antagonists (e.g. rimegepant, ubrogepant)
      6. Antiemetics (e.g. metoclopramide, prochlorperazine)
   B. Prophylactic therapy (frequent headaches, disrupted quality of life)
      1. Avoidance of triggers
      2. Lifestyle changes (e.g. good sleep hygiene, regular exercise)
      3. Beta blockers (e.g. propranolol, metoprolol)
      4. Antidepressants (e.g. amitriptyline, venlafaxine)
      5. Anticonvulsants (e.g. topiramate)
      6. CCBs (e.g. verapamil)
   C. Acute management of migraine in pregnancy
      1. Acetaminophen (first-line) or combination acetaminophen/metoclopramide
      2. Aspirin or NSAIDs (second-line)
      3. Ergots are contraindicated

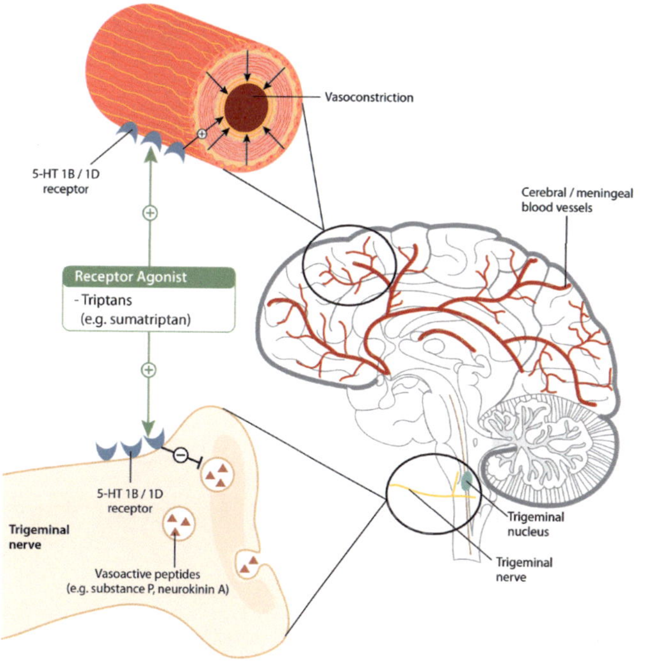

FIGURE 13.1.129 - Mechanism of Action of Triptans

VI. Cluster Headache: Definition
   A. Episodic severe primary headache disorder
   B. Often occurs in males

VII. Cluster Headache: Clinical Features
- A. Mostly unilateral, periorbital
- B. Duration: 15-180 minutes
- C. Daily attacks for few weeks followed by period of remissions
- D. Associated symptoms: autonomic (e.g. ipsilateral lacrimation, conjunctival injection, rhinorrhea, nasal congestion), agitation
- E. Ipsilateral ptosis and miosis may be present (partial Horner syndrome)
- F. Can be triggered by lack of sleep and alcohol

VIII. Cluster Headache: Diagnosis
- A. Mainly clinical
- B. Imaging (e.g. MRI) for first episode to rule out other conditions (e.g. brain lesions, Horner syndrome)

IX. Cluster Headache: Management
- A. Acute management
  1. High flow 100% oxygen
  2. Triptans (e.g. sumatriptan)
  3. Alternatives: ergots, lidocaine
- B. Prophylactic management
  1. Verapamil
  2. Topiramate

X. Tension Headache: Definition and Risk Factors
- A. Primary headache disorder
- B. Most prevalent type of headache
- C. Risk factors: fatigue, stress, anxiety, depression, lack of proper sleep

XI. Tension Headache: Clinical Features
- A. Bilateral
- B. Pain is mild-to-moderate, non-throbbing, constant, dull, and aching like a tight band around head
- C. Pericranial muscle tenderness
- D. Duration: 30 minutes to a week

XII. Tension Headache: Diagnosis
- A. Mainly clinical
- B. Imaging to rule out other conditions (e.g. brain lesions, giant cell arteritis)

XIII. Tension Headache: Management
- A. Avoid risk factors
- B. Massage
- C. Acute management
  1. NSAIDs (e.g. ibuprofen), acetaminophen, caffeine
- D. Prophylactic management
  1. TCAs like amitriptyline
  2. CBT, stress reduction techniques

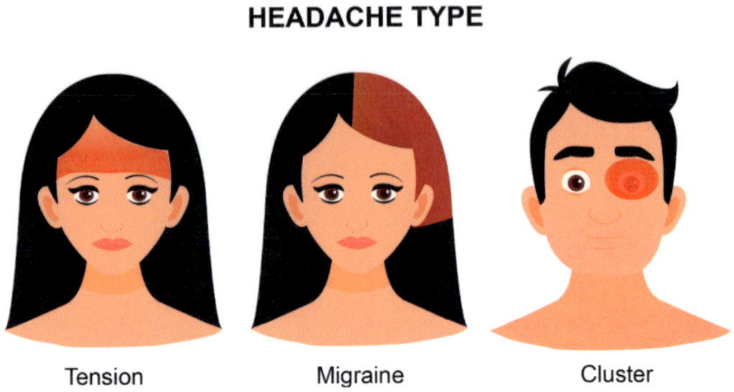

FIGURE 13.1.130 - Types of Primary Headache

XIV. Secondary Headache: Definition
- A. Headaches due to underlying medical condition or cranial pathology

XV. Secondary Headache: Causes
- A. Vascular (e.g. subarachnoid hemorrhage, subdural hematoma, epidural hematoma, temporal arteritis)
- B. Infectious (e.g. meningitis, encephalitis, cerebral abscess)
- C. Pharmacologic (e.g. nitrates, chronic analgesic use)
- D. Tumors or intracranial masses
- E. Other causes (e.g. hypertension, pseudotumor cerebri, pheochromocytoma)

XVI. Secondary Headache: Red Flags
- A. Sudden onset (seconds to minutes)
- B. New-onset in old age
- C. Change in mental status, signs of increased ICP (e.g. papilledema)
- D. Presence of seizures or focal neurologic symptoms/signs
- E. New-onset headache associated with
  1. Heavy exertion, head trauma
  2. Fever, neck stiffness, rash, HIV infection, cancer

XVII. Secondary Headache: Clinical Features, Workup, and Management
- A. Clinical presentations variable, depending upon the underlying cause (e.g. confusion, motor or sensory deficits)
- B. Workup: CBC, ESR, imaging (e.g. CT scan, MRI)
- C. Management: manage/correct the underlying cause

REVIEW QUESTIONS

1. A 25-year-old woman comes to her physician because of a severe headache that started 1 day ago. She states seeing flashing lights before the onset of the unilateral, pulsating headache. The patient asks the doctor to turn off the lights and close the window to block the traffic noise. This is her fifth episode of headache in the last 6 months. NSAIDs, acetaminophen, and antiemetics have not helped her previous episodes. What is the best next step in management?

   - **The best next step in management is to start a triptan such as sumatriptan to abort her migraines.**
   - This patient presents with a severe unilateral, pulsatile headache preceded by flashing lights. This description is consistent with a migraine headache with visual aura.
   - The patient asks the doctor to turn off the lights and close the window to block the traffic noise. This behavior is consistent with photophobia and phonophobia which further support the diagnosis of migraine headache.
   - NSAIDs, acetaminophen, and antiemetics have not helped her previous episodes, indicating escalation of treatment is necessary.

2. A 32-year-old man comes to the emergency department because of a severe headache that started half an hour ago. The headache is unilateral and most intense around the left eye. He states he experiences this type of headache every 3 months. Physical examination shows left-sided ptosis and anisocoria with a smaller left pupil. What two additional findings are also associated with this type of headache?

   - **Two additional findings that are also associated with cluster headaches include rhinorrhea and lacrimation.**
   - The patient presents with a severe unilateral headache that is most intense around the left eye. He experiences this roughly every 3 months.
   - Physical examination shows left-sided ptosis and anisocoria with a smaller left pupil.
   - These features are consistent with the diagnosis of a cluster headache.
   - Ptosis and miosis suggest a partial Horner syndrome that commonly accompanies the cluster headache.

3. A 62-year-old woman is brought to the emergency department by her son because of a severe headache and confusion. Her past medical history is significant for hypertension and migraines. On arrival she is alert and oriented only to self. Physical examination shows diffuse extremity weakness. What is the next best step in management?

   - **The best next step in management is to obtain an immediate non-contrast head CT scan.**
   - This patient is brought to the emergency department because of a severe headache associated with altered mental status.
   - Physical examination shows diffuse extremity weakness.
   - Although she has a history of migraine, her current headache with focal neurological deficits suggests a more ominous underlying cause such as a stroke. Therefore, the best next step is non-contrast head CT.

REVIEW QUESTIONS

4. A 21-year-old woman is brought to the emergency department by her roommate because of a progressively worsening right-sided headache associated with nausea and vomiting. The headache started 7 hours ago and was preceded by weakness of her left hand. Headache is described as unilateral, pulsating, and most intense around the right eye. She has had similar episodes in the past but have all been relieved with naproxen. She is under a lot of stress in college, and sometimes feels tension in her neck. Vital signs include temperature of 96.8° F (36° C), blood pressure of 110/75 mmHg, heart rate of 91 beats/min, and respiratory rate of 14 breaths/min. ESR and CRP are normal. Physical examination is unremarkable. She wants to lie in a dark silent room. Which of the following is the most likely cause of this patient's symptoms?

   A. Migraine headache
   B. Cluster headache
   C. Tension headache
   D. Temporal arteritis

- **The correct answer is option A.**
- This patient presents with a unilateral, pulsating headache associated with nausea and vomiting.
- The headache was preceded by weakness of her left hand, which is consistent with aura.
- She wants to lie in a dark silent room, which suggests photophobia and phonophobia.
- Considering that her vital signs and inflammatory markers are normal, all of these above findings are consistent with the diagnosis of the migraine headache.
- Option B is incorrect because cluster headache is a unilateral periorbital pain commonly associated with partial Horner syndrome, rhinorrhea, and lacrimation. Additionally, it is more common in males.
- Option C is incorrect because although this patient is under stress, and sometimes feels tension in her neck, this is not enough to diagnose her with the tension headache. Additionally, tension headaches are a bilateral headache not associated with nausea, vomiting, aura, photophobia, or phonophobia.
- Option D is incorrect. First, temporal arteritis is more common in elderly women. Second, it's commonly associated with jaw claudication and intermittent visual disturbances which are absent in this patient. The physical exam in the patient with temporal arteritis would have shown tenderness and a firm cord-like structure on the patient's lateral forehead.

Neurology | Section 27: Nervous System Tumors: Gliomas, Pilocytic Astrocytoma, GB Multiforme

I. Introduction: General Characteristics
   A. Primary brain tumors in adults
   B. 70% occur supratentorial
   C. Adults: glioblastoma multiforme, meningioma, ependymoma
   D. Primary brain tumors in children: second most common cancer
   E. 70% occur infratentorial
   F. Children: pilocytic astrocytoma, medulloblastoma
   G. Schwannomas: sporadically or neurofibromatosis

II. Introduction: Risk Factors
   A. Cigarette smoking
   B. Neurofibromatosis
   C. Turcot syndrome

III. Introduction: Clinical Features
   A. Headache: 20% initially, 60% later
   B. Tend to be worse during the night and often wakes the person up
   C. Visual disturbances
   D. Nausea and vomiting
   E. Seizures: > 30% of cases
   F. Impairment of balance, speech, hearing
   G. Personality or behavior changes

IV. Introduction: Imaging
   A. MRI with gadolinium enhancement
   B. CT scan: if calcium or hemorrhage is present
   C. Functional MRI: lesions in vital areas
   D. Positron emission tomography (PET)

V. Introduction: Treatment
   A. Surgery, irradiation, chemotherapy

VI. Gliomas: Definition
   A. Glial cells
   B. Cerebral hemispheres, brain stem
   C. Benign or malignant
   D. Grade I to IV
   E. Gliomas: Types/Grades
   F. Grade I and II: low grade
      1. Pilocytic astrocytoma (I)
      2. Diffuse astrocytomas (II)
   G. Grade III: diffuse, anaplastic astrocytoma
   H. Grade IV: glioblastoma

VII. Gliomas: Treatment
   A. Approach dependent on stage
   B. Grade I: watch and wait, surgery, radiation
   C. Grade II: surgical removal, radiation
   D. Grade III: chemotherapy, surgery, radiation
   E. Grade IV: surgery, radiation concurrent with chemotherapy

VIII. Pilocytic Astrocytoma: General Description
   A. Most common tumor CNS in children
   B. First two decades of life: 8-13 year olds
   C. Midline structures in posterior fossa
   D. Optic nerve (NF1), cerebellum

IX. Pilocytic Astrocytoma: Histology
   A. Rosenthal fibers
   B. Cysts

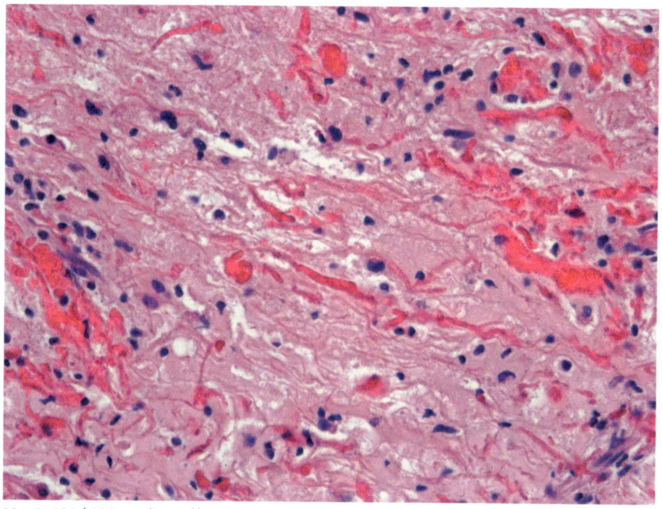

FIGURE 13.1.131 - Light Microscopy of Rosenthal Fibers in Pilocytic Astrocytoma

X. Pilocytic Astrocytoma: Imaging
   A. Cystic mass enhanced by contrast
   B. Mural nodule
   C. Calcifications

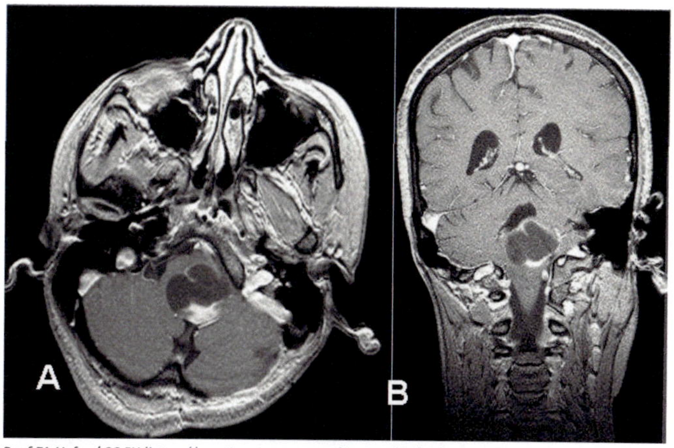

FIGURE 13.1.132 - MRI of the Brain: Pilocytic Astrocytoma

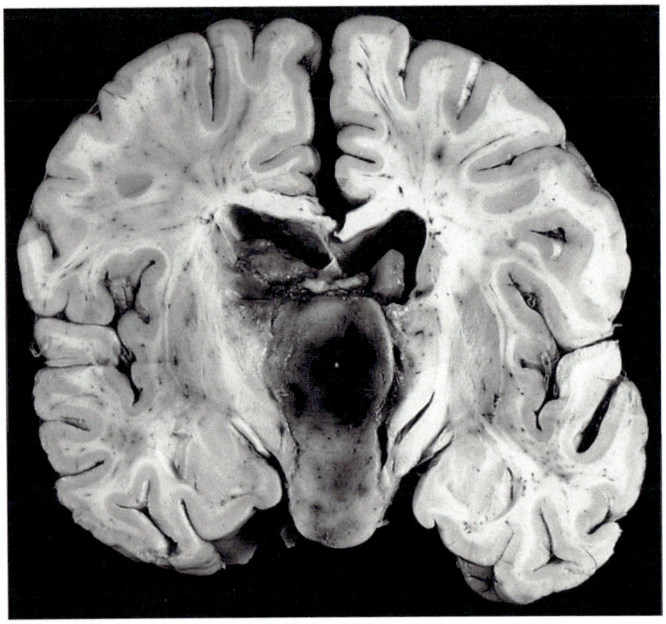

FIGURE 13.1.133 - Pilocytic Astrocytoma

XI. Pilocytic Astrocytoma: Prognosis
   A. 10 year survival is 100%: supratentorial and gross total resection

XII. Glioblastoma Multiforme: General Characteristics
   A. High-grade astrocytoma, stage IV glioma
   B. May arise de novo or from low grade astrocytoma
   C. Supratentorial
   D. IDH and 1p/19q codeletion
   E. Hemorrhagic tumor
      1. Multifocal areas of necrosis and cystic degeneration
      2. Commonly cross the corpus callosum

XIII. Glioblastoma Multiforme: Histology
   A. Marked anaplasia and pleomorphism
   B. Pseudopalisading necrosis
   C. GFAP, vimentin, S100

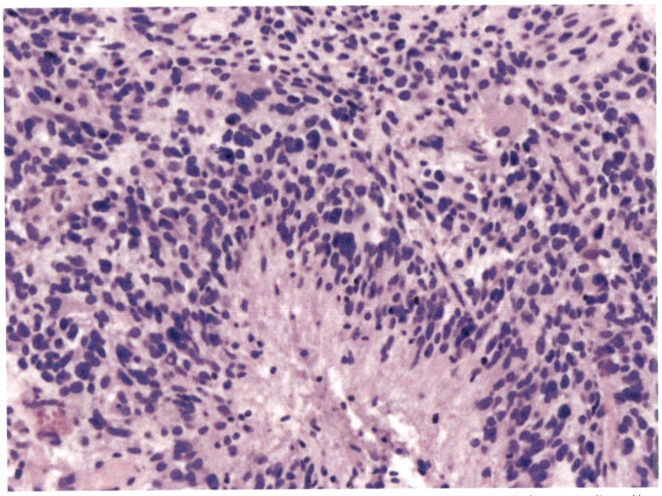

FIGURE 13.1.134 - Light Microscopy showing Pseudopalisading Necrosis in Glioblastoma Multiforme

XIV. Glioblastoma Multiforme: Imaging
   A. Large tumors
   B. Pseudocapsule
   C. Irregular thick margins, low density center
   D. Cross the corpus callosum

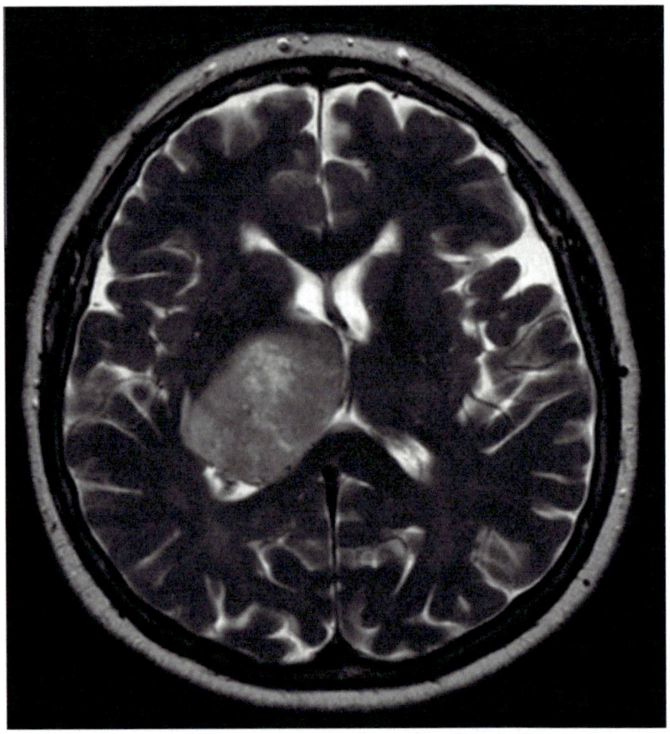

FIGURE 13.1.135 - MRI of the Brain: Glioblastoma Multiforme

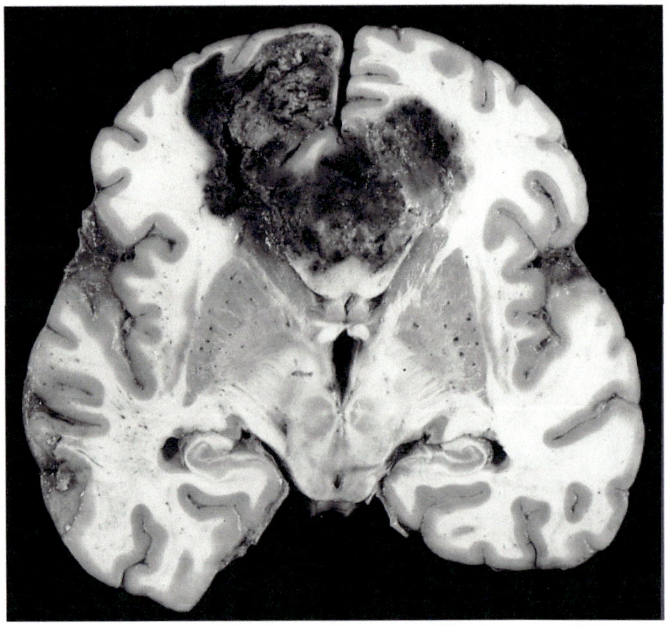

FIGURE 13.1.136 - Glioblastoma Multiforme

XV. Glioblastoma Multiforme: Prognosis
   A. Poor prognosis
   B. Death occurs in less than 1 year

REVIEW QUESTIONS

1. A 34-year-old woman comes to her primary care provider because of recurrent headaches over the last month. She says she has a history of tension migraines that typically occur in the middle of her work day and remit with over-the-counter pain medicines. Over the past month or so, her headaches have persisted despite pain medicines, and she says she occasionally gets woken up by headaches in the mornings. Review of systems is otherwise negative, and the physical examination is unremarkable. What is the next best step in management?

   - **The best next step in management of this patient is an MRI of the brain.**
   - This patient has a history of tension headaches
   - However, there is a new pattern for her headaches. Now, the headaches aren't improving with over the counter pain meds and wake her up from her sleep.
   - The next best step in this situation would be to order a brain MRI due to the pain pattern of her headaches, which could indicate malignancy.
   - There are two notable clues that suggest a brain tumor in this question stem: First her recent headaches no longer improve with pain medications. Second, she gets occasionally woken up by headaches.
   - A brain tumor should always be on the differential when patients report headaches that wake them up.

2. An 11-year-old boy is brought into the emergency department by his mother because of two weeks of worsening headaches and fatigue that have caused him to miss a lot of school. While in the emergency department, the boy vomits and becomes somnolent. An urgent MRI brain is ordered, and it shows a well-circumscribed mass compressing the cerebellum. What is the next best step in management?

   - **The next best step in management is a neurosurgery consultation.**
   - This child has been experiencing worsening headaches and fatigue.
   - MRI of the brain shows well-circumscribed mass compressing the cerebellum, which raises a suspicion of pilocytic astrocytoma.
   - Pilocytic astrocytomas are the most common benign pediatric brain tumors, and they typically originate around the cerebellum. They are considered to be grade I gliomas, which means that surgery can be curative.
   - Hence, the next step in management would be to consult neurosurgery for a potential surgical excision of this boy's brain tumor.

3. A 7-year-old girl is brought to the pediatrician by her dad because of concern for his daughter's vision over the last few weeks . Physical examination shows impaired vision in her right eye, brown spots in her iris bilaterally, and several hyperpigmented macules in her left axillary region. MRI of the brain and orbits is ordered, and shows a mass adjacent to the girl's right optic nerve. A biopsy of the mass reveals "stretched-out eosinophilic inclusions." What is the most likely diagnosis?

   - **The most likely diagnosis is optic glioma - neurofibromatosis type I.**
   - The girl has been experiencing impaired vision.
   - MRI of the brain and orbits shows a mass adjacent to the right optic nerve.
   - The biopsy of the mass shows "stretched-out eosinophilic inclusions," which is a common description of rosenthal fibers.
   - Therefore, this girl is most likely suffering from an optic glioma.
   - However, she also has several other findings on physical examination that are worth considering when deciding on the overarching diagnosis.
   - Specifically, the brown spots in her iris bilaterally are a description of Lisch nodules, and the several hyperpigmented macules in her left axillary region are a description of axillary freckling. Both Lisch nodules and axillary freckling are seen in patients with neurofibromatosis type I.
   - Hence, the most likely diagnosis in this case is a right-sided optic glioma in the setting of neurofibromatosis type I.

4. A clinician receives the biopsy results of her patient with a suspected glioma. The biopsy report describes marked anaplasia with pseudopalisading necrosis. The report also mentions that the tumor sample stained positive for GFAP. What is the grade of this patient's glioma?

   - **The patient's glioma is grade IV.**
   - Both grade I and grade IV gliomas can stain positive for GFAP, which makes this finding unhelpful in distinguishing them.
   - The histological finding of pseudopalisading necrosis, however, is a feature unique to glioblastoma multiforme.
   - Therefore, the most likely grade of this patient's glioma is a grade IV glioma or glioblastoma multiforme.

REVIEW QUESTIONS

5. A 55-year-old man comes to his primary care provider because of headaches for the past month. He says his headaches last for hours, do not resolve with pain medications, and often wake him up at night. Upon review of systems, he says he also lost about 10 lbs over the past two months. He is compliant with his medications. He is a chronic smoker, and denies alcohol use. Family history is unremarkable. His vital signs are within normal limits, along with the physical examination and full neurologic examination. A brain MRI reveals a heterogenous, poorly-demarcated mass that spans from the left parietal lobe to the right frontal lobe. What will the biopsy of the mass most likely show?

    A. Neoplastic cells with eosinophilic hair-like inclusions
    B. Marked anaplasia and pleomorphism with pseudopalisading necrosis
    C. Evenly distributed, uniform and rounded nuclei
    D. Monomorphic cells and perivascular pseudorosettes
    E. Interlacing bundles of elongated cells with palisading nuclei

- **The correct answer is option B.**
- This is a case of an older gentleman with worsening headaches.
- There are three clues that he may have brain cancer: First, his headaches wake him up at night. Second, he lost 10 lbs over the past two months. And third, he has a long-standing history of smoking.
- A brain MRI reveals a heterogenous, poorly-demarcated mass that spans from the left parietal lobe to the right frontal lobe. This description is consistent with glioblastoma multiforme. Additionally, glioblastoma multiforme should always be on the differential when suspecting a brain tumor in an older patient with a long-standing history of smoking because smoking is one of the key risk factors for development of brain tumors.
- Option A is incorrect because it describes rosenthal fibers, which are seen on biopsy of pilocytic astrocytomas. Pilocytic astrocytomas are grade I gliomas typically seen in children.
- Option C is incorrect because it describes the “fried-egg” appearance of cells seen in histology of oligodendroglioma. Oligodendrogliomas can be seen in adults, although they are more often well-circumscribed and homogenous on brain MRI and tend to be found in the frontal lobe.
- Option D is incorrect because it includes the buzz phrase “perivascular pseudorosettes” which are seen in cases of ependymomas. Ependymomas are more common in children and are usually seen around the 4th ventricle on brain MRI.
- Option E is incorrect because it describes the findings seen in Antoni A schwannomas. Schwannomas are most often located in the cerebellopontine angle on brain MRI.

Neurology | Section 28: Nervous System Tumors: Oligodendroglioma & Ependymoma

I. Oligodendroglioma: Definition
   A. Grade II glioma, derived from oligodendrocytes
   B. IDH mutation, codeletion (1p:19q)
   C. Middle age patients: more common in males
   D. Frontal lobe with frequent calcification

II. Oligodendroglioma: Histology
   A. Infiltrating mass
   B. Fried egg cell appearance
   C. Chicken wire pattern

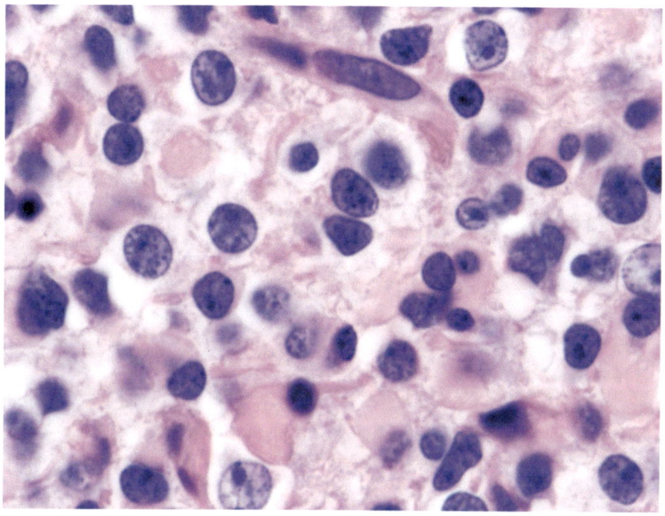

FIGURE 13.1.137 - Light Microscopy Showing Fried-Egg Appearance in Oligodendroglioma

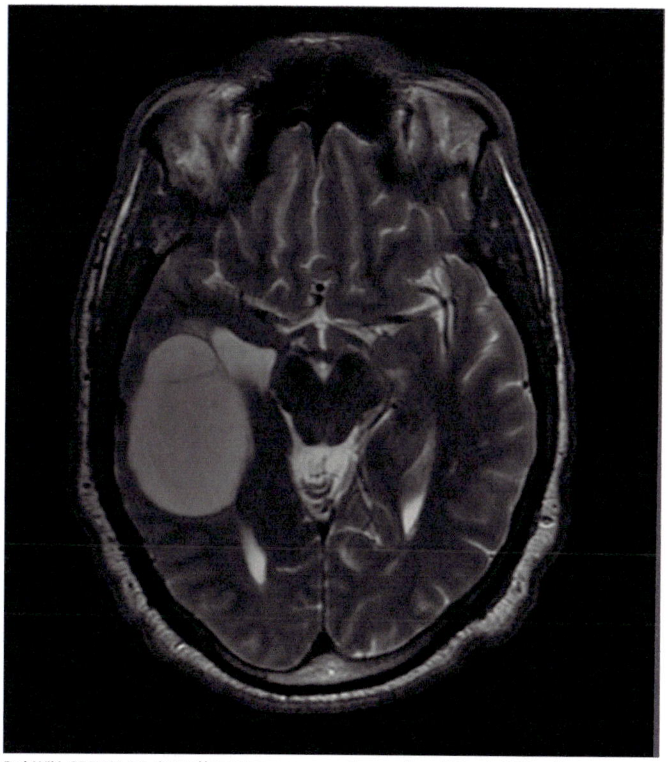

FIGURE 13.1.138 - MRI Displaying Oligodendroglioma

III. Ependymoma: General Characteristics
   A. Benign tumor derived from ependymal cells
   B. Infratentorial ependymomas: children
   C. Spinal tumors: adults
   D. Supratentorial ependymomas: both children and adults
   E. GFAP

IV. Ependymoma: Histology
   A. Monomorphic cells
   B. Perivascular pseudorosettes
   C. Calcifications, hyalinized vessels

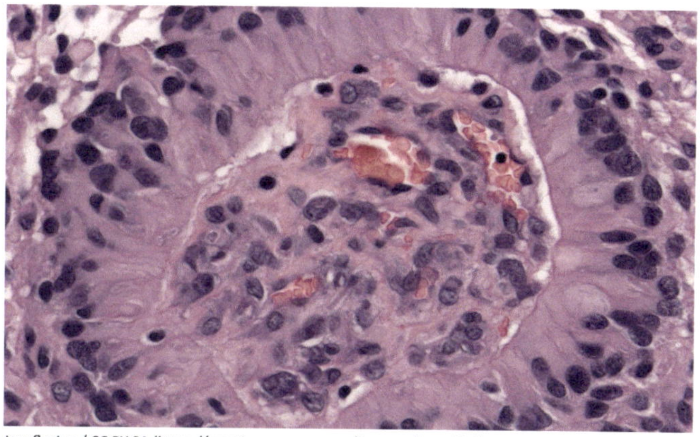

FIGURE 13.1.139 - Light Microscopy: Perivascular Pseudorosettes in Ependymoma

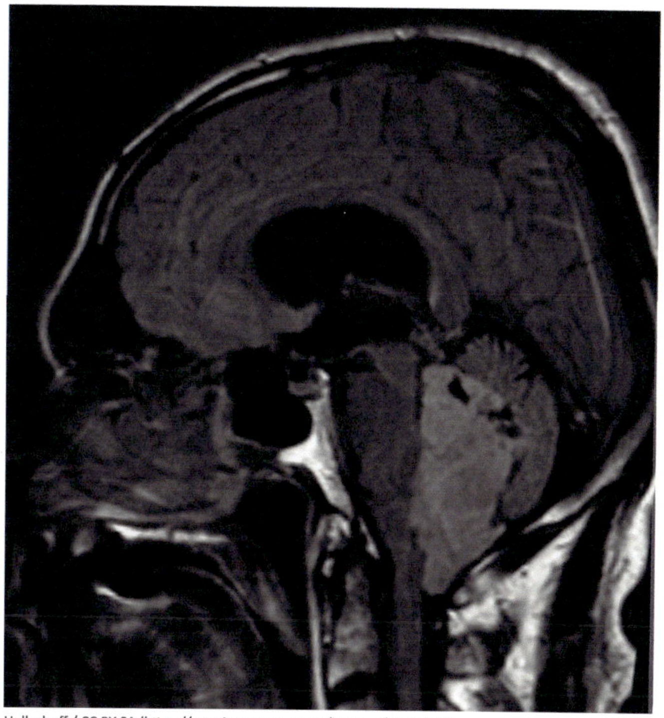

FIGURE 13.1.140 - MRI of the Brain: Ependymoma

V. Ependymoma: Prognosis
   A. Good prognosis

REVIEW QUESTIONS

1. What symptoms would you expect in a patient with an oligodendroglioma in the left frontal lobe?
    - **Symptoms expected in a patient with an oligodendroglioma in the left frontal lobe include personality changes and difficulties in speech.**
    - One of the most unique sets of symptoms that manifest as a result of masses in the frontal lobe are sudden and dramatic personality changes. Patients may become uncharacteristically irritable, impulsive, or aggressive. Some may lose their social awareness or even exhibit social disinhibition in the form of behaviors in public that are not deemed appropriate.
    - Broca's area is located in the left frontal lobe in the majority of people, and it is responsible for articulation and production of speech. Hence, people with masses in the left frontal lobe may report difficulties with speech.

2. What is a common risk factor for development of ependymomas in the pediatric population?
    - **In the pediatric population, a common risk factor for development of ependymomas is neurofibromatosis type 2.**
    - This is in contrast to pilocytic astrocytomas and optic gliomas, which are traditionally associated with neurofibromatosis type 1.

Neurology | Section 29: Schwannoma, Medulloblastoma, Hemangioblastoma

I. Schwannoma: Definition
   A. Benign tumor derived from Schwann cells
   B. CN V and CN VIII may be involved
   C. Neurofibromatosis type 2
   D. Acoustic neuromas
      1. CN VIII
      2. Cerebellopontine angle
      3. Encapsulated tumors, unilateral

II. Schwannoma: Clinical Features
   A. Associated with neurofibromatosis (NF2)
      1. Usually bilateral tumors
   B. Tinnitus
   C. Sensorineural deafness
   D. Sensory changes in CN V distribution
      1. Due to tumor impingement on CN V

III. Schwannoma: Histology
   A. Antoni A: interlacing bundles of elongated cells with palisading nuclei
   B. Antoni B: looser, less cellular pattern than Antoni A

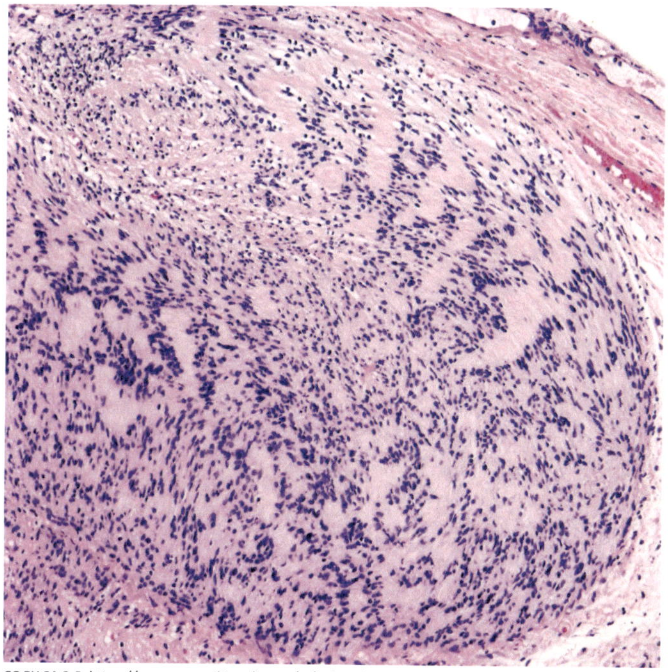

FIGURE 13.1.141 - Light Microscopy: Antoni A Pattern in Schwannoma

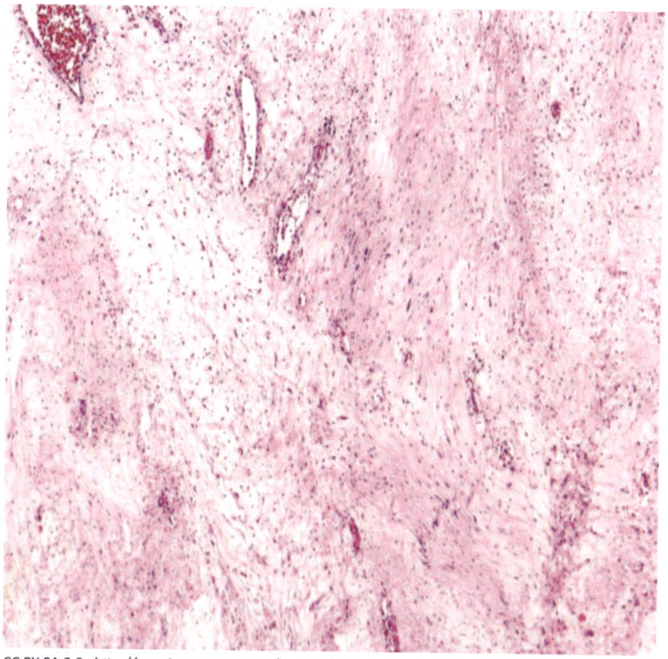

FIGURE 13.1.142 - Light Microscopy: Antoni B Pattern in Schwannoma

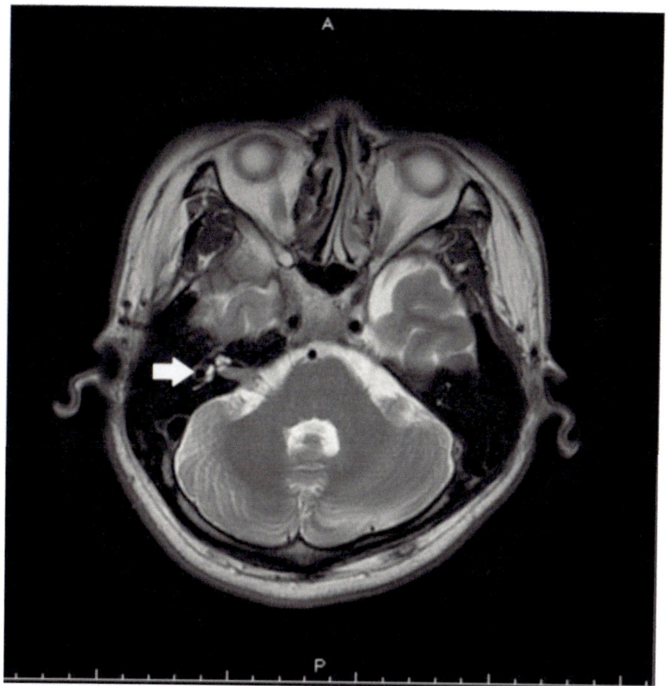

FIGURE 13.1.143 - MRI of the Brain: Schwannoma

IV. Schwannoma: Prognosis
   A. Good prognosis
   B. Surgery required

V. Medulloblastoma: Definition
   A. Malignant small cell tumor: primitive neuroectodermal tumor
   B. Primarily occurs in children

VI. Medulloblastoma: Clinical Features
   A. Mass effect, hydrocephalus
   B. Cerebellum involvement: ataxia, wide based gait
   C. Often seeds the neuraxis and invades the fourth ventricle
   D. Cerebrospinal fluid pathways

VII. Medulloblastoma: Diagnosis
   A. Sheets of closely packed small blue cells
   B. Scant cytoplasm
   C. Arranged in rosette or perivascular pseudorosette pattern
      1. Homer Wright rosette

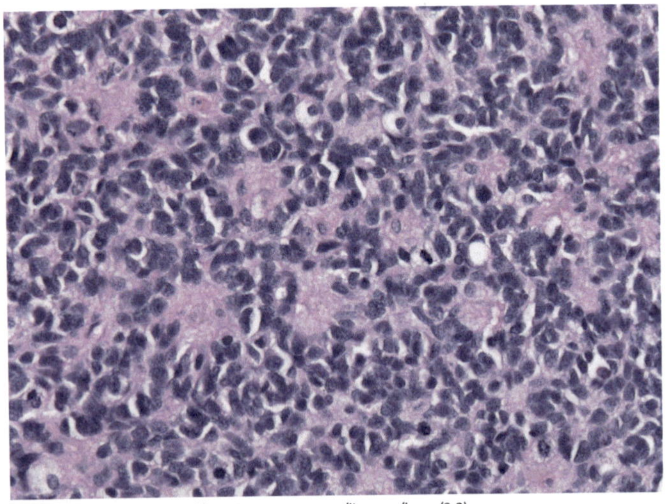

FIGURE 13.1.144 - Light Microscopy: Homer Wright Rosettes in Medulloblastoma

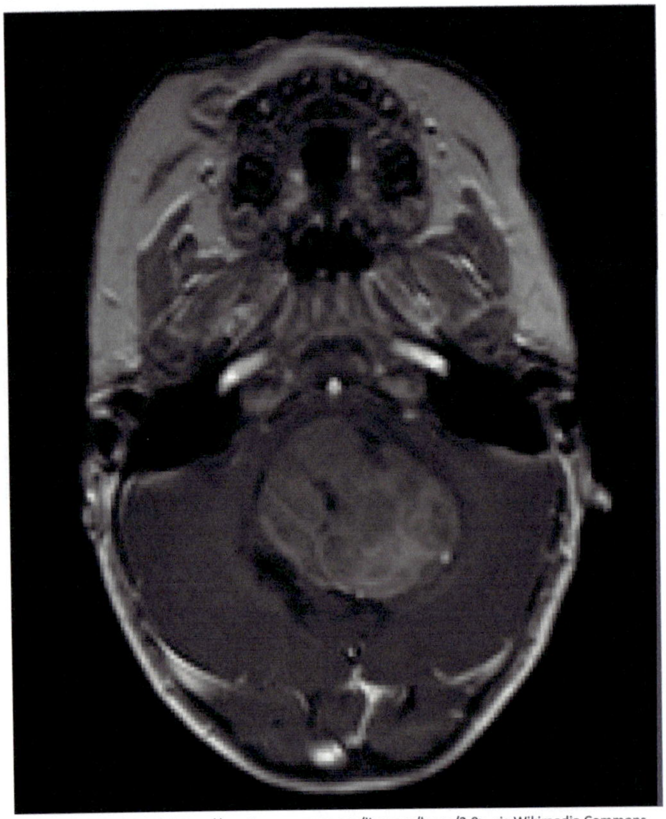

FIGURE 13.1.145 - MRI of the Brain: Medulloblastoma

VIII. Medulloblastoma: Treatment
   A. Radiosensitive: most effective postoperative treatment
   B. Poor prognosis
   C. *P53* mutation: worst prognosis

IX. Hemangioblastoma: Definition
   A. Most frequently in the posterior fossa
   B. Von Hippel Lindau
      1. Hemangioblastomas
      2. Renal cell carcinoma
      3. Pheochromocytomas

X. Hemangioblastoma: Clinical Features
   A. Depend on location and growth
   B. Cerebellum: ataxia, discoordination, mass effect
   C. Ocular or systemic symptoms

XI. Hemangioblastoma: Diagnosis
   A. Proliferation of capillaries
   B. Disorganized arrangement
   C. PAS+ lipid
   D. Pleomorphic stromal cells

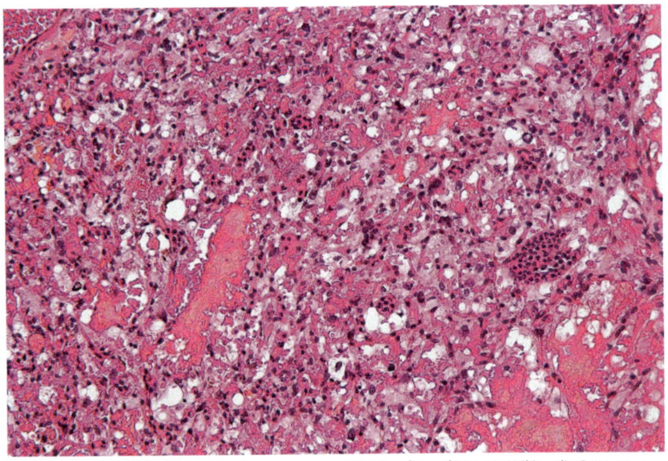

FIGURE 13.1.146 - Light Microscopy: Hemangioblastoma

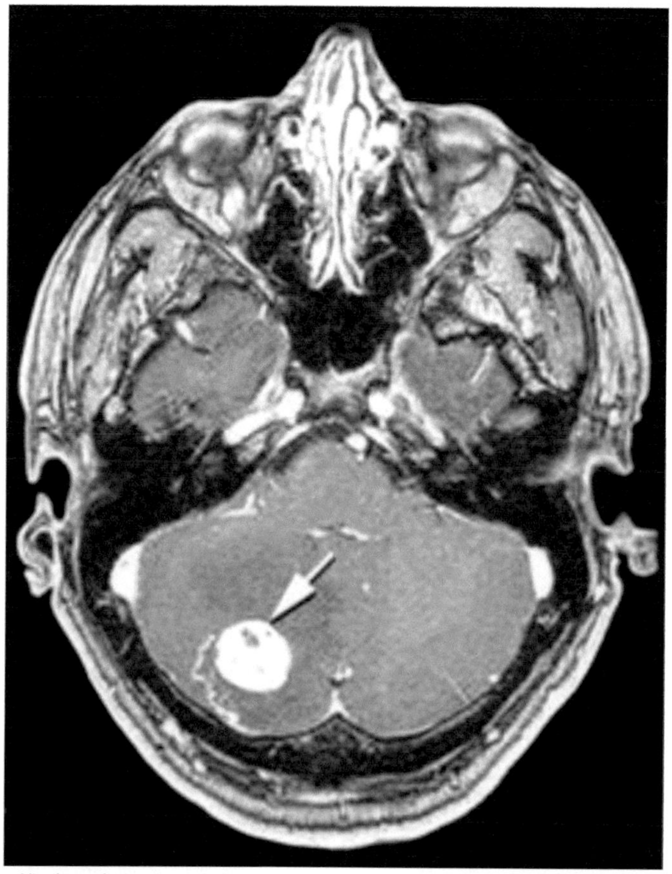

FIGURE 13.1.147 - MRI of the Brain: Hemangioblastoma

REVIEW QUESTIONS

1. A 21-year-old man with known medulloblastoma visits his primary care physician for routine follow up and is scheduled for a screening colonoscopy due to a family history of colon cancer. The colonoscopy reveals hundreds of polyps within the colon. What is the most likely underlying diagnosis?
   - **The most likely diagnosis is Turcot syndrome.**
   - This syndrome is characterized by familial adenomatous polyposis, cafe au lait spots, and CNS tumors, such as medulloblastoma.

2. A patient was recently diagnosed with a hemangioblastoma and the clinician suspects this patient may have von Hippel-Lindau syndrome. What other malignancies would warrant diagnostic consideration?
   - **Other malignancies that would warrant diagnostic consideration include central nervous system and retinal hemangioblastomas, clear cell renal cell carcinoma, and pheochromocytoma.**
   - Von Hippel-Lindau syndrome is a multisystemic tumor predisposition syndrome characterized by benign and malignant tumors, including central nervous system (CNS) and retinal hemangioblastomas, clear cell renal cell carcinoma (RCC), and pheochromocytoma.
   - A useful mnemonic to remember about von Hippel-Lindau is HARP.
   - "H" stands for hemangioblastoma.
   - "A" stands for angiomatosis.
   - "R" stands for renal cell carcinoma.
   - "P" stands for pheochromocytoma.

Neurology | Section 30: Meningioma, Sellar & Suprasellar Tumor & Secondary Brain Tumors

I. Meningioma: Definition
   A. Arachnoid cells
   B. Most common benign CNS tumor in adults

II. Meningioma: Clinical Features
   A. Female predominance: estrogen, progesterone receptors
   B. Neurofibromatosis type 2
   C. History of radiation
   D. Seizures
   E. Hearing loss
   F. Anosmia

III. Meningioma: Diagnosis
   A. Swirling masses of meningothelial cells encompass psammoma bodies (calcified bodies)

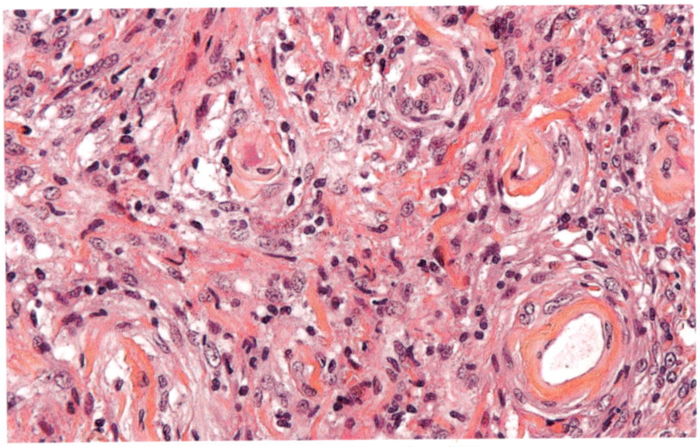

FIGURE 13.1.148 - Light Microscopy: Psammoma Body in Meningioma

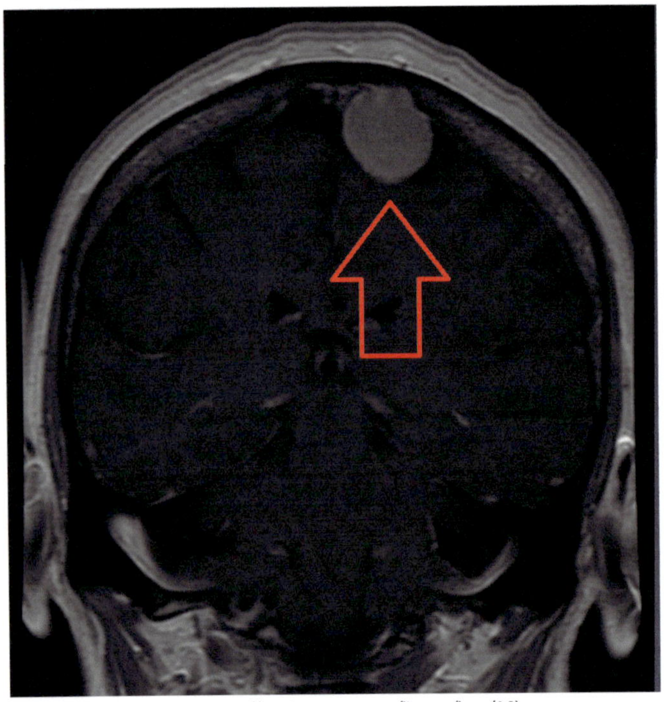

FIGURE 13.1.149 - MRI of the Brain: Meningioma

IV. Sellar and Suprasellar Tumors: Definition
   A. Pituitary adenomas: sellar
   B. Benign tumors anterior pituitary
   C. Suprasellar tumors: extend to neighboring structures (sphenoid sinus, cerebellopontine angle, pineal region)
   D. Craniopharyngiomas: sellar or suprasellar
   E. Remnants of Rathke's pouch

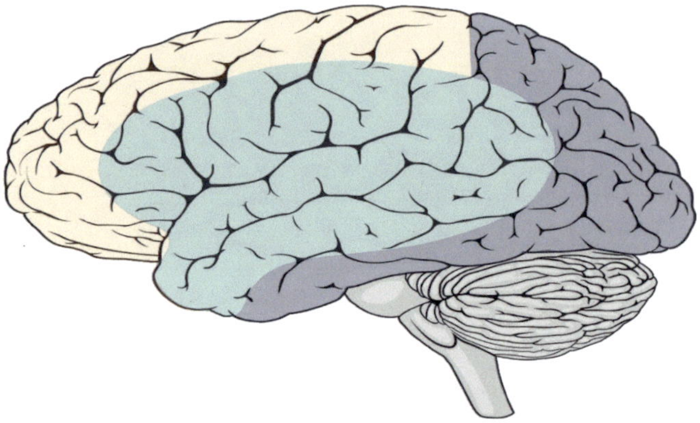

FIGURE 13.1.150 - The Pituitary Gland

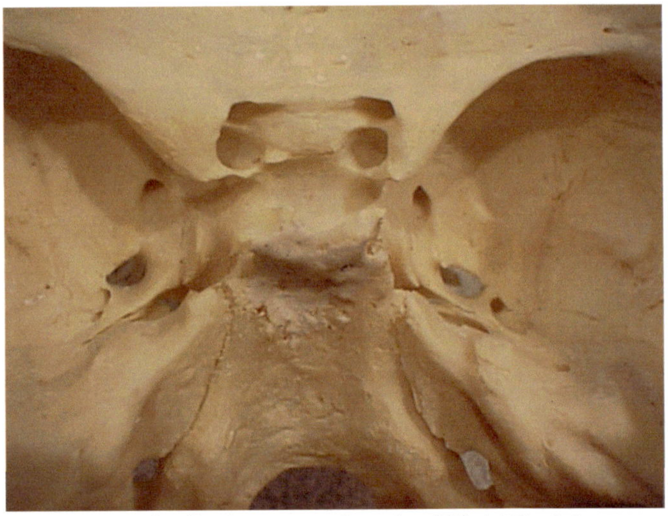

FIGURE 13.1.151 - The Sella Turcica

V. Sellar and Suprasellar Tumors: Clinical Features
   A. Pituitary adenomas: functional or non-functional
      1. Nonfunctional: mass effect
      2. Headaches, hypopituitarism
      3. Prolactinomas, growth hormone, ACTH, TSH, LH, FSH
   B. Craniopharyngiomas
      1. Present in bimodal age distribution:
         a) Children: 5-14 years old
         b) Adults: 50-74 years old
      2. Calcifications commonly seen
      3. Benign but tend to recur after resection
      4. Mass effect
      5. Supratentorial mass compressing optic chiasm

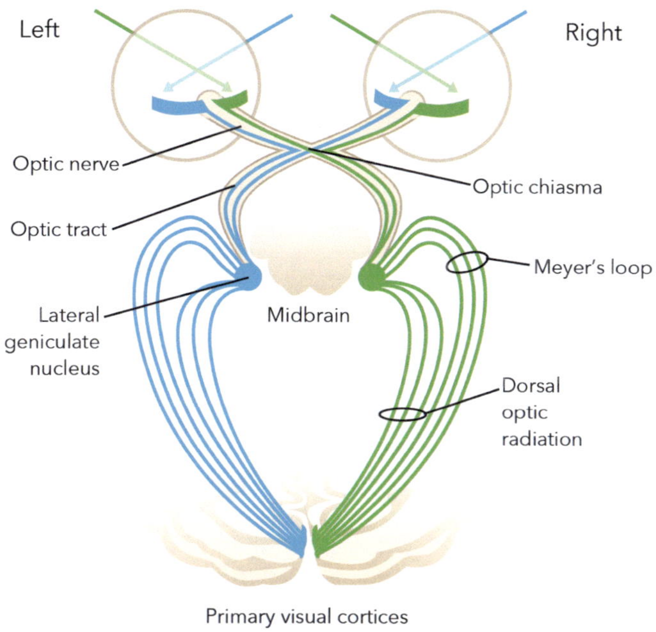

FIGURE 13.1.152 - The Optic Pathway

VI. Sellar and Suprasellar Tumors: Diagnosis
   A. Abundant cytoplasm
   B. Cytoplasmic appearance usually correlates with content of hormone containing secretory cells
   C. Craniopharyngiomas
      1. Sheets of compact cells
      2. Yellow fluid rich in cholesterol crystals

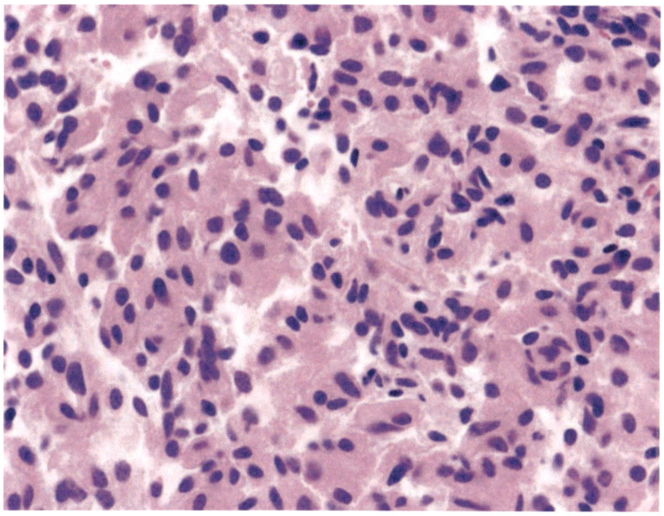

FIGURE 13.1.153 - Light Microscopy: Cells of Pituitary Adenoma

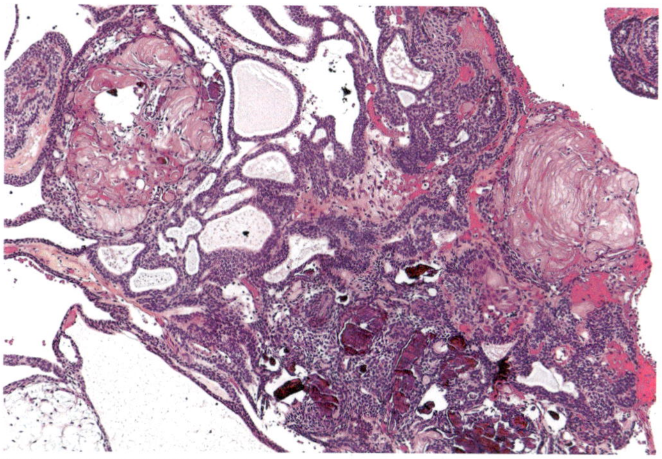

FIGURE 13.1.154 - Light Microscopy: Craniopharyngioma

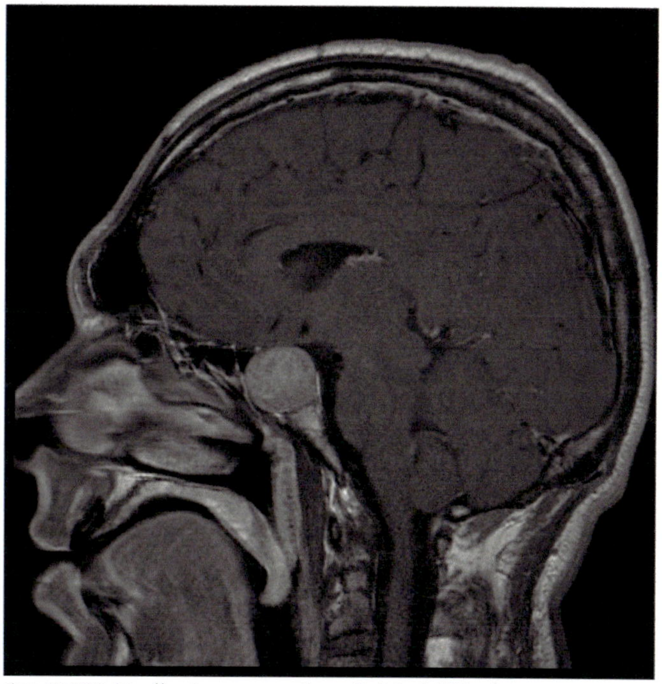

FIGURE 13.1.155 - MRI of the Brain: Pituitary Adenoma

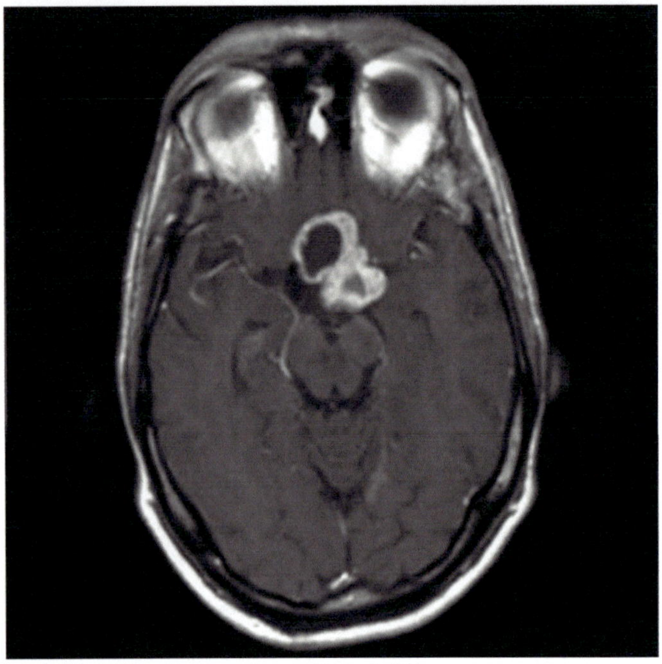

FIGURE 13.1.156 - MRI of the Brain: Craniopharyngioma

VII. Metastatic Brain Tumors: Definition
   A. More common than any primary neoplasm
   B. Multiple, well circumscribed lesions: at gray-white junction
   C. Originate from primary sites: lung, breast, melanoma, kidney, GI
   D. Existing malignancy, stage/grade
   E. More common in adults

VIII. Metastatic Brain Tumors: Clinical Features
   A. Increased intracranial pressure
   B. Headache
      1. Worsens when lying down
      2. Localized or diffuse
      3. "Head in a vise"
      4. Dull, piercing, throbbing
   C. Vomiting, seizures, alteration in consciousness

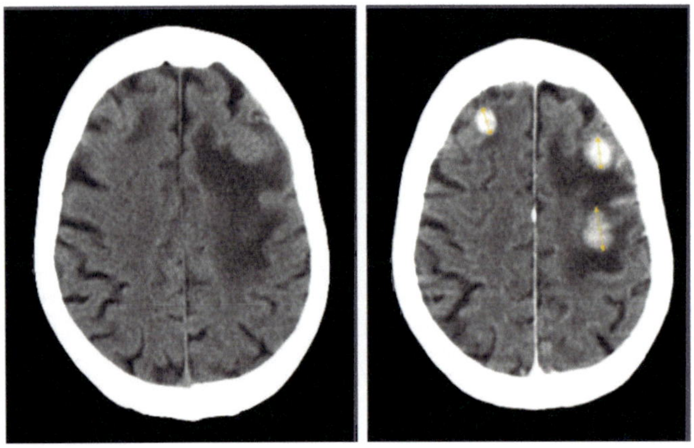

FIGURE 13.1.157 - CT Scan of the Head: Metastatic Brain Tumors

IX. Metastatic Brain Tumors: Treatment
   A. Non-chemotherapeutic drugs
   B. Chemotherapy avoided: absent blood-brain barrier diffusion capacity
   C. Surgery, radiation

REVIEW QUESTIONS

1. Aside from meningioma, which other cancers may exhibit psammoma bodies on histologic examination?
   - **Other cancers that may exhibit psammoma bodies on histologic examination are mesothelioma, papillary thyroid carcinoma, serous papillary endometrial carcinoma, and serous papillary ovarian carcinoma.**

2. What signs and symptoms would be expected in a male patient with a prolactinoma?
   - **Signs and symptoms in a male patient with prolactinoma are erectile dysfunction, decreased libido, and occasionally gynecomastia.**
   - Normally, prolactin inhibits GnRH and sex hormone secretion. It also promotes breast growth. Therefore, elevated levels of prolactin can cause erectile dysfunction, decreased libido, and occasionally gynecomastia.

3. What features of a headache should prompt suspicion for an underlying brain tumor?
   - **Features of a headache that should prompt suspicion for an underlying brain tumor are headaches upon awakening or headaches that no longer respond to treatment.**
   - Headaches caused by brain tumors are often so severe that they wake patients up at night or are worse in the morning, due to the increased intracranial pressure and mass effect.
   - In patients with a history of headaches, if a headache suddenly becomes different and no longer responds to treatments that were known to work in the past, a clinician should consider the possibility of a brain tumor.

REVIEW QUESTIONS

4. A 66-year-old woman with a history of tension headaches comes to her primary care provider because of worsening headaches occurring for the last 5 days. She says her current headaches have been worse than usual, do not resolve to pain medications, and have been waking her up from sleep. Her past medical history is notable for hypertension and hyperlipidemia. Patient has been smoking one pack of cigarettes daily for the past 40 years. Vital signs are notable only for elevated blood pressure. Physical examination, including a full neurologic examination, was unremarkable. Review of records indicates a lung mass was found on a prior screening which the patient never followed-up on. A MRI of the brain is ordered. Which of the following findings will likely be seen on imaging?

    A. A midline mass in the fourth ventricle
    B. A sharply demarcated homogenous mass with a cystic wall and a mural nodule
    C. A homogenous parasagittal mass with a dural tail
    D. A hyperdense mass in the sellar region
    E. Multiple cannonball lesions at the gray-white junction

- **The correct answer is option E.**
- The patient is at high risk of having brain cancer.
- She reports a history of worsening headaches that no longer remit with pain medications and wake her up from sleep. This should immediately prompt suspicion of a brain tumor.
- She reports a 40-pack year smoking history and her records are notable for a lung mass that she never followed-up on. This should raise suspicion for an undiagnosed lung cancer.
- Putting the two clues together, this patient likely has brain metastases from her underlying lung cancer.
- Therefore, the correct option will be one that describes what brain metastases typically look like on brain MRI, and that is option E.
- Option A is incorrect because a midline mass in the fourth ventricle is more suggestive of a medulloblastoma. In general, medulloblastomas are more commonly seen in children rather than adults.
- Option B is incorrect because a sharply demarcated homogenous mass with a cystic wall and a mural nodule is more suggestive of a hemangioblastoma. Hemangioblastomas can be associated with Von Hippel-Lindau syndrome.
- Option C is incorrect because a homogenous parasagittal mass with a dural tail is a classic description of a meningioma. Meningiomas are the most common benign brain tumors in adults and tend to occur more frequently in women than men. Given the likely history of lung cancer in this patient, a meningioma is less likely than brain metastases.
- Option D is incorrect because a hyperdense mass in the sellar region is a finding consistent with suprasellar tumors, such as a pituitary adenoma or a craniopharyngioma. Either of these brain tumors is less likely in the context of this patient's presumed lung cancer.

Neurology | Section 31: Dizziness & Vertigo

I. Central Vertigo: Introduction
   A. Dizziness
      1. Vertigo: sensation of spinning while being stationary
      2. Presyncope: actual imbalance due to decreased cerebral perfusion

II. Central Vertigo: Definition
   A. Sensation of spinning while being stationary due to central nervous system dysfunction

III. Central Vertigo: Causes
   A. Vestibular migraine
   B. Cerebellar/brainstem stroke
   C. Multiple sclerosis
   D. Intracranial tumors

IV. Central Vertigo: Clinical Presentation
   A. General features
      1. Nystagmus (oscillatory eye movements) with any direction
         a) Fast & slow phase, named based on direction of fast phase
         b) Non-fatigable (lasts more than 1 minute) and not inhibited by gaze fixation on the object
         c) No latency period (time between provocative test and the onset of nystagmus)
      2. No tinnitus or hearing loss
      3. CNS symptoms (e.g. diplopia, dysarthria, numbness, weakness)
      4. Walking not preserved
   B. Vestibular migraine
      1. Vertigo with nystagmus
      2. Vertigo is absent between the migraine episodes
      3. Other migraine features (e.g. unilateral pulsating headache, photophobia)
   C. Multiple sclerosis
      1. CNS demyelinating disorder
      2. Vertigo with nystagmus
      3. Other features of multiple sclerosis (e.g. optic neuritis, spastic weakness, neurogenic bladder)
   D. Cerebellar stroke
      1. Sudden-onset, persistent vertigo
      2. Other cerebellar signs (e.g. ataxia, dysmetria, dysdiadochokinesia)
   E. Brainstem stroke
      1. Sudden-onset, persistent vertigo
      2. Contralateral sensory/motor loss; ipsilateral cranial nerve deficit
   F. Intracranial tumor
      1. Mostly infratentorial tumors cause vertigo with nystagmus (e.g. cerebellar hemangioblastoma)
      2. Other symptoms depend on the exact location and may include
         a) Seizures
         b) Sensory loss and motor weakness
         c) Dysarthria and dysphagia

V. Central Vertigo: Diagnosis
   A. Brain imaging
      1. MRI or CT scan depending on suspected etiology
   B. Caloric test
      1. Warm water in the ear canal causes ipsilateral nystagmus
      2. Cold water in the ear canal causes contralateral nystagmus
      3. Abnormal results: unilateral/bilateral weakness (peripheral disease), failure of fixation suppression (central disease)

VI. Central Vertigo: Management
   A. Antiemetics, antihistamines, antimuscarinics to prevent vomiting
   B. Treat the underlying condition
      1. Vestibular migraine: sumatriptan or dihydroergotamine
      2. Multiple sclerosis: multifactorial therapy (e.g. natalizumab, baclofen, IV steroids)
      3. Stroke: aspirin, clopidogrel, tPA (ischemic stroke)
      4. Intracranial tumor: surgery, chemoradiotherapy, or both

VII. Peripheral Vertigo: Definition
   A. Sensation of spinning while being stationary due to dysfunction of inner ear or vestibulocochlear nerve

VIII. Peripheral Vertigo: Pathophysiology
   A. Inner ear or vestibulocochlear nerve dysfunction sends abnormal impulses to the vestibular system
   B. Examples
      1. Benign paroxysmal positional vertigo
      2. Vestibular neuritis; acute labyrinthitis
      3. Meniere disease
      4. Acoustic neuroma

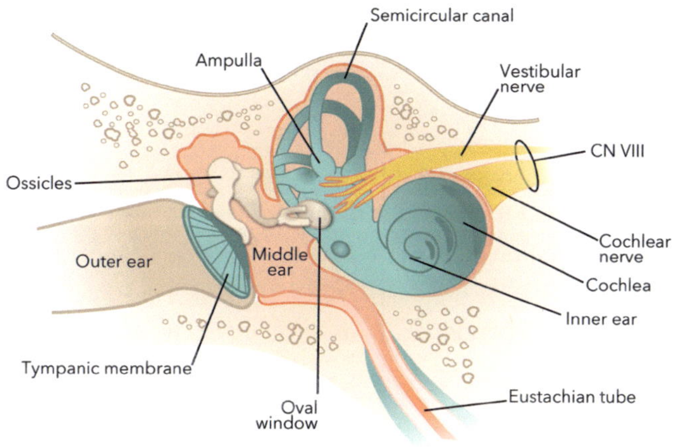

FIGURE 13.1.158 - Inner Ear

IX. Peripheral Vertigo: Clinical Presentation
- A. General features
  1. Nystagmus
     - a) Mostly horizontal; never purely vertical or purely torsional
     - b) Fatigable (lasts less than 1 minute)
     - c) Inhibited by gaze fixation on the object
     - d) Latency period up to 1 minute
  2. Possible hearing loss and tinnitus
  3. No other CNS symptoms
  4. Walking preserved
- B. Benign paroxysmal positional vertigo (BPPV)
  1. Displaced otoliths in semicircular canals
  2. Vertigo induced by rotating head movements (e.g. turning in bed) and backward head tilt
  3. Brief episodes (seconds to minutes) of vertigo +/- nystagmus
  4. No auditory symptoms (e.g. tinnitus, hearing loss)
- C. Vestibular neuritis
  1. Inflammation of the vestibular nerve
  2. Associated with current or previous viral infection
  3. Episode of vertigo can last for days
  4. No hearing loss
- D. Labyrinthitis
  1. Symptoms of vestibular neuritis and hearing loss
- E. Meniere disease
  1. Endolymphatic hydrops: accumulation of endolymph in the inner ear
  2. Triad of vertigo + tinnitus (ringing in the ears) + sensorineural hearing loss
- F. Acoustic neuroma (vestibular schwannoma)
  1. Schwann cell tumor arising from the cranial nerve VIII
  2. Mostly unilateral tumor in the cerebellopontine angle
  3. Bilateral tumors associated with neurofibromatosis type II
  4. Vertigo and sensorineural hearing loss
  5. Bell's palsy (CN VII); decreased facial sensation (CN V), ataxia (cerebellum)

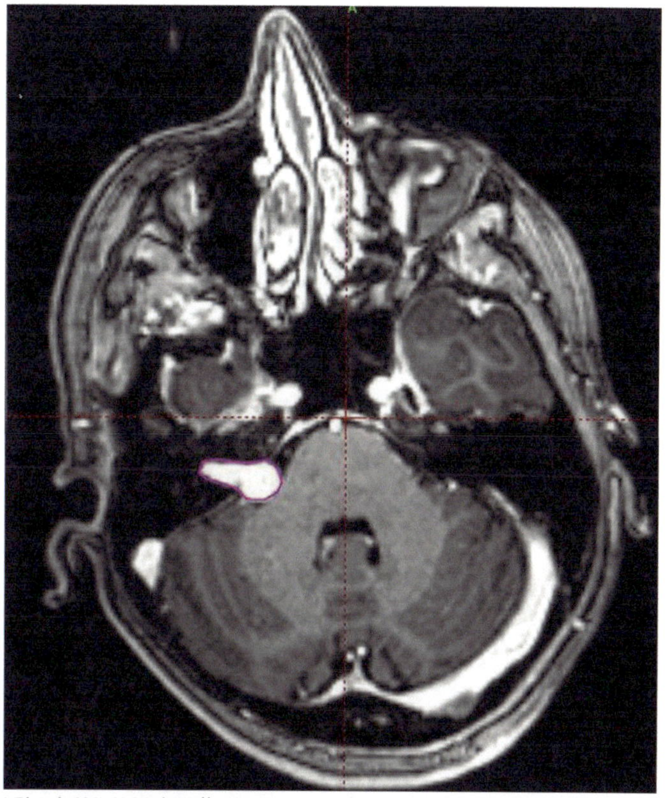

FIGURE 13.1.159 - MRI of the Brain: Acoustic Neuroma

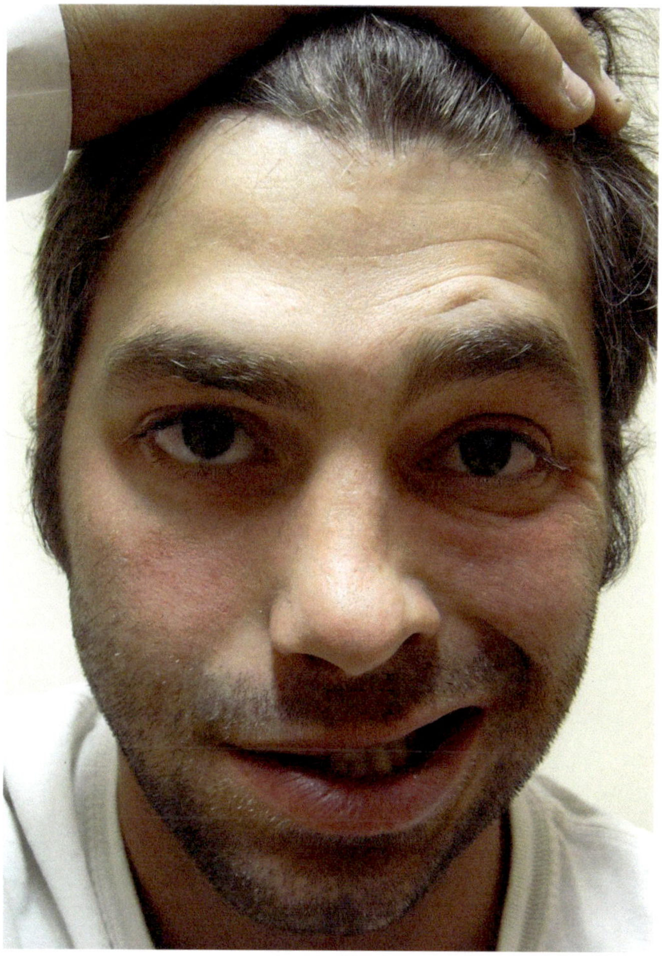

FIGURE 13.1.160 - Bell's Palsy

X. Peripheral Vertigo: Diagnosis
   A. BPPV: Dix-Hallpike maneuver
   B. Audiometry
   C. MRI of the brain
   D. Head thrust test

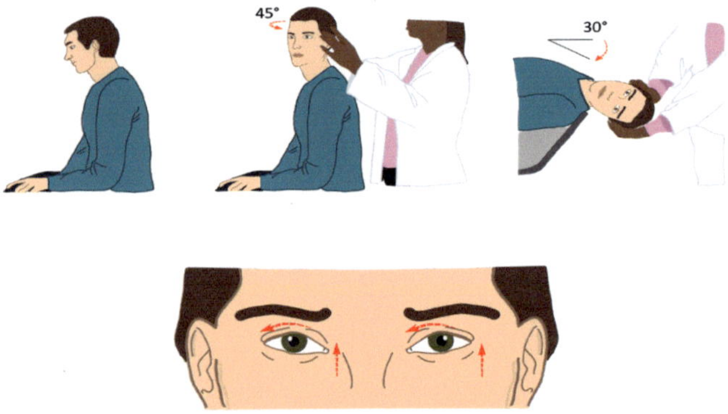

FIGURE 13.1.161 - Dix-Hallpike Maneuver

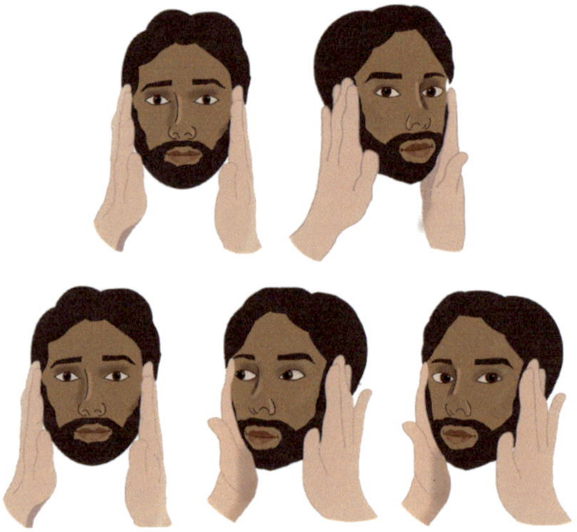

FIGURE 13.1.162 - Head Thrust Test

XI. Peripheral Vertigo: Management
   A. Antiemetics, antihistamines, antimuscarinics to prevent vomiting
   B. Cause-specific management
      1. BPPV: Epley maneuver
      2. Vestibular neuritis: acyclovir is herpes simplex virus is suspected
      3. Labyrinthitis: consider oral corticosteroids
      4. Meniere disease: low-salt diet and diuretics
      5. Acoustic neuroma: surgical excision

Central Vertigo	Peripheral Vertigo
- Nystagmus in any direction	- Mostly horizontal nystagmus - Never purely vertical or purely torsional
- Non-fatigable (lasts more than 1 minute)	- Fatigable (lasts less than 1 minute)
- Not inhibited by gaze fixation on object	- Inhibited by gaze fixation on object
- No latency period	- Latency period up to 1 minute
- No hearing loss or tinnitus	- Hearing loss or tinnitus
- Other CNS symptoms	- Usually no other CNS symptoms
- Walking usually not preserved	- Walking preserved

TABLE 13.1.16 - Types of Vertigo

Causes of Vertigo	Key Features
Vestibular migraine	- Typical features of migraine - Vertigo with nystagmus during migraine attack - No vertigo in between attacks
Multiple sclerosis	- Vertigo with nystagmu - Optic neuritis, spasticity, neurogenic bladder, vertigo with nystagmus
Cerebellar/ brainstem stroke	- Focal neurological deficits - Vertigo with nystagmus
Intracranial tumor	- Focal neurological deficits - Seizures - Vertigo with nystagmus
BPPV	- Displaced otoliths in semicircular canals - Diagnosed with Dix-Hallpike maneuver - Treated with Epley maneuver
Vestibular neuritis	- Post-viral vertigo lasting for days - No hearing loss
Acute labyrinthitis	- Post-viral vertigo lasting for days with hearing loss
Meniere disease	- Endolymphatic hydrops - Triad: vertigo, tinnitus, and hearing loss
Acoustic neuroma	- Cerebellopontine angle tumor - Bilateral acoustic neuroma associated with neurofibromatosis type II

TABLE 13.1.17 - Causes of Vertigo

REVIEW QUESTIONS

1. A 65-year-old man is brought to the emergency department because of a severe headache that started 2 hours ago. His past medical history is significant for uncontrolled hypertension. Physical exam shows left-sided dysmetria and dysdiadochokinesia. The patient feels dizzy and he has oscillatory eye movements with the fast phase to the left. A Non-contrast CT scan of the head shows a hypodense area in the left cerebellum. What are the most likely characteristics to describe this patient's eye movements?
   - **The most likely characteristic to describe this patient's eye movements, in a case of central vertigo, is that the nystagmus is non-fatigable with no latency period. Additionally, it is not inhibited by gaze fixation, and it is not associated with hearing loss or tinnitus.**
   - This patient has a severe acute headache.
   - He has a history of uncontrolled hypertension.
   - The physical exam shows left-sided dysmetria and dysdiadochokinesia.
   - Non-contrast head CT scan reveals hypodense area in the left cerebellum.
   - All of these findings are consistent with an ischemic cerebellar stroke.
   - He feels dizzy, and he has oscillatory eye movements with the fast phase to the left. This is the classic description of vertigo with nystagmus.
   - Since he has the cerebellar stroke, he likely has central vertigo.
   - Patients with central vertigo commonly have other CNS symptoms like dysmetria, dysdiadochokinesia, or dysarthria.

2. A 35-year-old woman is brought to the emergency department because of sudden left-sided vision loss and pain in her left eye for the last 3 hours. She also complains of urinary incontinence. She had weakness of her left hand 2 weeks ago and paresthesia on her right thigh 4 weeks ago, but these symptoms have completely resolved. Physical exam shows vertical upbeating nystagmus. What is the best next step in the management of this patient?
   - **The next best step in the management of this patient is to obtain a MRI of the brain.**
   - This young woman has sudden vision loss and a painful left eye. This is likely consistent with optic neuritis.
   - She had weakness in her left hand 2 weeks ago and paresthesia on her right thigh 4 weeks ago.
   - This description is consistent with the symptoms disseminated in time and space. In other words, the patient experiences symptoms on different parts of her body during different times.
   - She also complains of urinary incontinence.
   - The physical exam shows vertical upbeat nystagmus.
   - All of these findings suggest the diagnosis of multiple sclerosis.
   - The best next step in the diagnosis of multiple sclerosis is MRI of the brain to look for the areas of demyelination.

REVIEW QUESTIONS

3. A 27-year-old woman comes to her primary care provider because of recurrent episodes of dizziness for the last 6 months. During an episode she feels like the room is spinning around her. These episodes last seconds to minutes, and she experiences the symptoms when she turns her head rapidly to the side. Looking up also triggers her episodes. Caloric test induces oscillatory eye movements. What are the most likely characteristics to describe this patient's eye movements?

   - **In a case of peripheral vertigo, the most likely characteristics of eye movement is that the nystagmus is never purely vertical or purely torsional. Additionally, it's fatigable, and it is inhibited by gaze fixation. It has a latency period, and is associated with hearing loss or tinnitus.**
   - This patient presents with brief episodes of vertigo.
   - The episodes last seconds to minutes, and she experiences the symptoms when she turns from side to side in bed. Looking up also triggers her episodes.
   - This is the classic description of the benign paroxysmal positional vertigo, that is, BPPV.
   - Caloric test induces oscillatory eye movements, or nystagmus.
   - BPPV is the cause of peripheral vertigo.
   - The other CNS symptoms are usually absent.

4. A 40-year-old man comes to his primary care physician due to left-sided hearing loss for the last 3 weeks.. He also reports hearing a ringing sound in his left ear, and states he has episodes where he feels like the room is spinning around him, causing him to vomit. His wife has noticed oscillatory movements of his eyes whenever he feels dizzy. Audiometry confirms sensorineural hearing loss. In addition to antiemetic medications, which two interventions will likely benefit this patient?

   - **Two interventions that will likely benefit this patient are salt restriction and diuretics.**
   - This patient has sensorineural hearing loss, tinnitus, and vertigo accompanied by nystagmus. This triad is consistent with the diagnosis of Meniere disease.
   - Meniere disease is caused by endolymphatic hydrops, that is, accumulation of excess endolymph within the scala media of the labyrinth.
   - In addition to antiemetic medications, patients with Meniere disease typically benefit from low-salt diet and diuretics which decrease the endolymph production.

Neurology | Section 32: Syncope

I. Syncope: Definition
   A. Loss of consciousness due to decreased cerebral perfusion

II. Syncope: Pathophysiology
   A. Decreased cerebral perfusion due to
      1. Decreased blood volume (hypovolemia)
         a) Diarrhea, vomiting, intensive perspiration, bleeding
      2. Vagus nerve activation
         a) Vasovagal syncope
      3. Hypersensitive carotid sinus
      4. Autonomic neuropathy
         a) Diabetes mellitus, Parkinson's disease
      5. Tachyarrhythmias
         a) Ventricular tachycardia/fibrillation, SVT
      6. Bradyarrhythmias
         a) Sick sinus syndrome, sinus bradycardia, AV block

III. Syncope: Clinical Presentation
   A. Hypovolemia
      1. Sunken eyes
      2. Dry skin and mucous membranes
      3. Decreased skin turgor (skin tenting)
   B. Vasovagal (neurocardiogenic) syncope
      1. Triggered by stress and prolonged standing
      2. Prodromal diaphoresis
      3. Warmth
      4. Nausea
      5. Pallor
      6. Rapid regain of consciousness
   C. Carotid hypersensitivity
      1. Sudden syncope with tactile stimulation of carotid sinus (e.g. shaving, tight collar)
      2. Rapid regain of consciousness
   D. Autonomic neuropathy
      1. Syncope while rapidly standing from supine or seated position
      2. Other signs of underlying condition
         a) Hyperglycemia in diabetes
         b) Motor deficits in Parkinson's disease
   E. Tachyarrhythmias (cardiogenic syncope)
      1. Palpitations
      2. Sudden onset with no warning signs or symptoms
      3. ECG abnormalities specific to the arrhythmia
   F. Bradyarrhythmias (cardiogenic syncope)
      1. Preexisting fatigue
      2. Preexisting dyspnea on exertion
      3. Palpitations
      4. Prodrome with lightheadedness
      5. ECG abnormalities (e.g. sinus arrest, sinus block, dropped QRS)

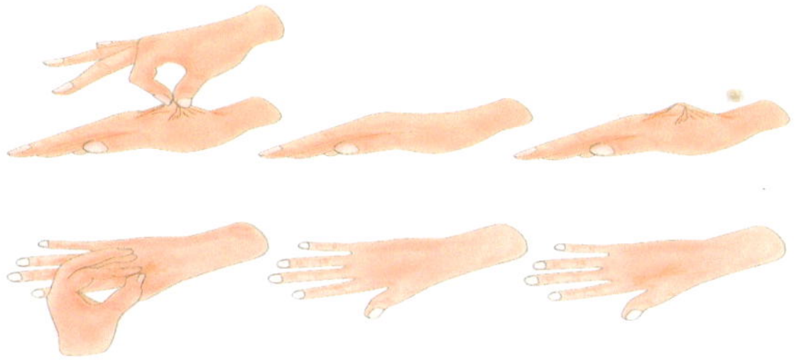

FIGURE 13.1.163 - Decreased Skin Turgor

IV. Syncope: Diagnosis
   A. Hypovolemia: vital signs measurement (hypotension, tachycardia)
   B. Vasovagal syncope: clinical diagnosis; upright tilt table test
   C. Carotid hypersensitivity: patient history and syncope during carotid massage
   D. Autonomic neuropathy: history, physical exam and blood glucose measurement
   E. Arrhythmias: ECG (e.g. wide QRS, fibrillatory waves, sinus block)

V. Syncope: Management
   A. Hypovolemia: fluid resuscitation
   B. Vasovagal syncope: avoidance of triggers; counter-pressure techniques (e.g. crossing the legs, arm tensing, squeeze rubber ball)
   C. Carotid hypersensitivity: avoidance of triggers
   D. Autonomic neuropathy: treatment of underlying condition
   E. Arrhythmias: antiarrhythmic medications; synchronized and unsynchronized cardioversion

Causes of Syncope	Key Features
Hypovolemia	- Diarrhea, vomiting - Intensive perspiration - Bleeding
Vasovagal syncope	- Vagus nerve overactivity - Triggered by prolonged standing or stress - Prodrome (diaphoresis, pallor)
Carotid hypersensitivity	- Tactile stimulation of carotid sinus (e.g. shaving, tight collar)
Autonomic neuropathy	- Diabetes mellitus - Parkinson's disease
Tachyarrhythmias	- Palpitations - Sudden onset with no warning signs
Bradyarrhythmias	- Palpitations - Prodrome with lightheadedness

TABLE 13.1.18 - Causes of Syncope

REVIEW QUESTIONS

1. A 36-year-old man comes to the primary care physician because of two episodes of fainting for the past month. Both episodes occurred when he was shaving. He cannot wear a necktie because it makes him feel "dizzy." What is the most likely pathophysiology causing this patient's loss of consciousness?

   - **The most likely pathophysiology of loss of consciousness in this patient is external pressure is applied to the carotid sinus, the vagus nerve gets overactive, and it decreases the heart rate. Decreased heart rate lowers the cardiac output and cerebral perfusion resulting in syncope.**
   - This patient had two episodes of fainting, and both episodes occurred when he was shaving. Additionally, he cannot wear a necktie because it makes him feel "dizzy."
   - These findings are consistent with the diagnosis of syncope due to carotid sinus hypersensitivity.
   - In this condition, carotid sinus baroreceptors are hypersensitive to external pressure on the neck such as necktie, or tight collar.
   - External pressure on carotid sinus → vagus nerve overactivation → ↓ heart rate and cardiac output → ↓ cerebral perfusion→ syncope.

2. A 55-year-old woman comes to the primary care physician because of 3 episodes of fainting in the past 4 months. Her past medical history includes Hashimoto thyroiditis for 20 years, type II diabetes mellitus for 2 years, and paroxysmal supraventricular tachycardia self-treated with carotid sinus massage. Her fainting episodes have no precipitating factor but are preceded by lightheadedness and fatigue. Physical exam shows dry skin and brittle hair and nails. Resting ECG shows no abnormalities. Vital signs include blood pressure of 120/80 mmHg, heart rate of 48 beats/min, and respiratory rate of 14 breaths/min in the supine position. When she stands up, her blood pressure becomes 115/78 mmHg, and the heart rate increases to 65 beats/min but she does not feel dizzy. Her TSH is 10 mIU/L (0.5-5.0 mIU/L). Which of the following is the most likely cause of this patient's occasional loss of consciousness?

   A. Cardiogenic syncope
   B. Neurocardiogenic syncope
   C. Autonomic neuropathy
   D. Carotid hypersensitivity

- **The correct answer is option A.**
- This patient presents with 3 episodes of fainting.
- She has a long-term history of Hashimoto thyroiditis.
- She has dry skin and brittle hair and nails.
- Her resting heart rate is 48 beats/min, and her resting ECG is normal.
- Her TSH is 10 mIU/L.
- This is consistent with poorly controlled hypothyroidism.
- She has a sinus bradycardia likely due to hypothyroidism.
- Sinus bradycardia decreases cardiac output and cerebral perfusion resulting in syncope. Therefore, the most likely cause of occasional loss of consciousness in this patient is cardiogenic syncope.
- Option B, neurocardiogenic or vasovagal syncope, is incorrect because this patient's fainting episodes have no precipitating factor, unlike vasovagal syncope which is triggered by stress or prolonged standing.
- Option C, autonomic neuropathy, is incorrect because this patient has a very short-term history of diabetes mellitus. Additionally, standing up causes normal hemodynamic changes in this patient suggesting that her autonomic nervous system functions normally.
- Option D, carotid hypersensitivity, is incorrect because this patient's fainting episodes are not triggered by external pressure on the carotid sinus.

TABLES & FIGURES

TABLE 13.1.1 - Types of Stroke....7
TABLE 13.1.2 - CHA2DS2-VASc Score....9
TABLE 13.1.3 - Brain Death, Coma, and Vegetative State....37
TABLE 13.1.4 - Glasgow Coma Scale....37
TABLE 13.1.5 - MG vs LEMS....47
TABLE 13.1.6 - Duchenne Muscular Dystrophy vs. Becker Muscular Dystrophy....48
TABLE 13.1.7 - Neurofibromatosis Type I, Neurofibromatosis Type II, and Tuberous Sclerosis....52
TABLE 13.1.8 - Sturge-Weber Syndrome and Von-Hippel-Lindau Disease....55
TABLE 13.1.9 - Types of Seizures....66
TABLE 13.1.10 - Types of Seizures....67
TABLE 13.1.11 - Differential Diagnosis of Seizures....69
TABLE 13.1.12 - Aphasia, Neglect, Gerstmann's Syndrome, Agnosia, and Apraxia....73
TABLE 13.1.13 - Localization of Cortical and Subcortical Lesions....76
TABLE 13.1.14 - Localization of Brainstem Lesions....77
TABLE 13.1.15 - Classic Spinal Cord Lesions....80
TABLE 13.1.16 - Types of Vertigo....110
TABLE 13.1.17 - Causes of Vertigo....110
TABLE 13.1.18 - Causes of Syncope....113
FIGURE 13.1.1 - The Cerebral Homunculus....7
FIGURE 13.1.2 - The Deep Brain Structures....7
FIGURE 13.1.3 - CT Scan of the Head: Ischemic Stroke....8
FIGURE 13.1.4 - MRI of the Brain: Ischemic Stroke....8
FIGURE 13.1.5 - ECG: Atrial Fibrillation....8
FIGURE 13.1.6 - Management of Stroke....9
FIGURE 13.1.7 - The Danger Triangle....12
FIGURE 13.1.8 - The Cavernous Sinus....12
FIGURE 13.1.9 - Horner Syndrome....12
FIGURE 13.1.10 - MR Venography: Cerebral Venous Thrombosis....13
FIGURE 13.1.11 - CT Scan of Head: "Empty Delta" Sign....13
FIGURE 13.1.12 - Parkinson Disease....15
FIGURE 13.1.13 - Livedo Reticularis....16
FIGURE 13.1.14 - MRI of Brain: Atrophy of Caudate Nucleus....16
FIGURE 13.1.15 - Friedreich Ataxia....19
FIGURE 13.1.16 - Hammer Toes....19
FIGURE 13.1.17 - Conjunctival Telangiectasia....19
FIGURE 13.1.18 - Meninges....23
FIGURE 13.1.19 - Kernig Sign....23
FIGURE 13.1.20 - Brudzinski Sign....23
FIGURE 13.1.21 - Light Microscopy of Gram Stained CSF Sample: Gram-Negative Diplococci....23
FIGURE 13.1.22 - Petechiae and Purpura....23
FIGURE 13.1.26 - Diagnosis and Management of Meningitis....24
FIGURE 13.1.27 - Purulent CSF Sample....25
FIGURE 13.1.28 - MRI of the Brain: Temporal Lobe Hyperintensity in HSV Encephalitis....26
FIGURE 13.1.29 - MRI of the Brain: Brain Abscess....27
FIGURE 13.1.30 - Spinal Epidural Abscess....28
FIGURE 13.1.31 - MRI of the Spinal Cord: Spinal Epidural Abscess....28
FIGURE 13.1.32 - Healthy Brain vs. Brain in Severe Alzheimer's Dementia....30
FIGURE 13.1.33 - Light Microscopy: Senile Plaques in Alzheimer's Dementia....30
FIGURE 13.1.34 - Light Microscopy: Neurofibrillary Tangles in Alzheimer's Dementia....30
FIGURE 13.1.35 - CT Scan of the Brain: Multiple Hypodensities in Periventricular and Subcortical White Matter and Basal Ganglia in Vascular Dementia....30
FIGURE 31.1.36 - MRI of the Brain: Atrophy of Frontal and Temporal Lobes in Frontotemporal Dementia....31
FIGURE 13.1.37 - Light Microscopy: Pick Bodie....31
FIGURE 13.1.38 - Enlarged Ventricles and Atrophy of Temporal Lobe in Frontotemporal Dementia....31
FIGURE 13.1.39 - Light Microscopy: Lewy Body....31

FIGURE 13.1.40 - MRI of the Brain: Enlarged Ventricles in Normal Pressure Hydrocephalus....32
FIGURE 13.1.41 - Light Microscopy: Spongiform Changes in Creutzfeldt-Jakob Disease....32
FIGURE 13.1.42 - MRI of the Brain: Hyperintense Signals in the Cortex and Basal Ganglia in Creutzfeldt-Jakob Disease....32
FIGURE 13.1.43 - Mini Mental State Examination....33
FIGURE 13.1.44 - Mechanism of Action of Certain Medications....33
FIGURE 13.1.45 - Types of Brain Herniation....37
FIGURE 14.1.46 - Lateral Positioning....37
FIGURE 13.1.47 - MRI of the Head: Glioma....38
FIGURE 13.1.48 - Lumbar Puncture....38
FIGURE 13.1.49 - Features of Alcohol Withdrawal....39
FIGURE 13.1.50 - Neuron Structure....41
FIGURE 13.1.51 - Right Internuclear Ophthalmoplegia....41
FIGURE 13.1.52 - MRI of the Brain: Multiple Demyelinating Plaques in Multiple Sclerosis....42
FIGURE 13.1.53 - MRI of the Brain: Demyelination in Progressive Multifocal Leukoencephalopathy....42
FIGURE 13.1.54 - Neuromuscular Junction....45
FIGURE 13.1.55 - Pathophysiology of Myasthenia Gravis....45
FIGURE 13.5.56 - Ptosis and Strabismus in Myasthenia Gravis....46
FIGURE 13.5.57 - Myasthenia Gravis vs. Lambert-Eaton Myasthenic Syndrome....46
FIGURE 13.5.58 - Pseudohypertrophy of Calf Muscles....47
FIGURE 13.1.59 - Light Microscopy Replacement of Muscle Tissue by Adipose Tissue in DMD....48
FIGURE 13.1.60 - Cafe-Au-Lait Spots....50
FIGURE 13.1.61 - Cutaneous Neurofibromas....50
FIGURE 13.1.62 - Lisch Nodules....50
FIGURE 13.1.63 - Brushfield Spots....50
FIGURE 13.1.64 - MRI of the Brain: Optic Glioma....50
FIGURE 13.1.65 - MRI of the Brain: Bilateral Acoustic Neuromas....51
FIGURE 13.1.66 - Cataracts....51
FIGURE 13.1.67- Facial Angiofibromas....51
FIGURE 13.1.68 - Ash-Leaf Spot....52
FIGURE 13.1.69 - Echocardiography: Cardiac Rhabdomyoma....52
FIGURE 13.1.70 - MRI of the Abdomen: Bilateral Renal Angiomyolipomas....52
FIGURE 13.1.71 - Ungual Fibroma....52
FIGURE 13.1.72 - Port-Wine Stain....54
FIGURE 13.1.73 - CT Scan of Head: Leptomeningeal Angiomas with Calcifications....54
FIGURE 13.1.74 - MRI of the Brain and Spinal Cord: Hemangioblastomas....54
FIGURE 13.1.75 - Renal Cell Carcinoma....55
FIGURE 13.1.76 - Pheochromocytoma....55
FIGURE 13.1.77 - Cross-Section of the Spinal Cord: Area Affected in Anterior Cord Syndrome....57
FIGURE 13.1.78 - Anterior Spinal Artery....57
FIGURE 13.1.79 - Cross-Section of the Spinal Cord: Area Affected in Central Cord Syndrome....57
FIGURE 13.1.80 - Cross-Section of the Spinal Cord: Area Affected in Brown-Sequard Syndrome....58
FIGURE 13.1.81 - Brown-Sequard Syndrome....58
FIGURE 13.1.82 - Spinal Canal and Cauda Equina....60
FIGURE 13.1.83 - MRI of Lumbosacral Spine....60
FIGURE 13.1.84- Cross Section of the Spinal Cord with a Human Outline....61
FIGURE 13.1.85 - Syringomyelia....61
FIGURE 13.1.86 - Spinal MRI: Transverse Myelitis....61
FIGURE 13.1.87 - Oculosympathetic Pathway....63
Figure 13.1.88 - Miosis and Ptosis in a Patient with Horner Syndrome....63
FIGURE 13.1.89 - Pancoast Tumor on Chest X-Ray....64
FIGURE 13.1.90 - Types of Seizures....66
FIGURE 13.1.91 - EEG: Generalized 3 Hz Spike-Wave Discharge in Absence Seizures....67
FIGURE 13.1.92 - Anatomy of the Brain....72
FIGURE 13.1.93 - Blood Supply to Different Areas of the Brain....72
FIGURE 13.1.94 - Broca Area, Wernicke Area and Arcuate Fasciculus....72
FIGURE 13.1.95 - A Clock Drawn by a Person with Neglect....73
FIGURE 13.1.96 - Area Affected in Gerstmann's Syndrome....73
FIGURE 13.1.97 - The Corticospinal Tract....75
FIGURE 13.1.98 - Spinothalamic Tract....75
FIGURE 13.1.99 - Dorsal Column-Medial Lemniscus Pathway....75
FIGURE 13.1.100 - Lateral Side of Cerebral Hemisphere....76
FIGURE 13.1.101 - The Homunculus....76
FIGURE 13.1.102 - The Optic Pathway....76

FIGURE 13.1.103 - Conjugate Eye Deviation Towards Lesion Side....77
FIGURE 13.1.104- CT Scan of the Head: Lacunar Infarcts....77
FIGURE 13.1.105 - Cross-Section of Medulla Oblongata: Area Affected in Medial Medullary Syndrome....77
FIGURE 13.1.106 - Cross-Section of Medulla Oblongata: Area Affected in Lateral Medullary Syndrome....78
FIGURE 13.1.107 - Cross-Section of the Pons: Area Affected in Lateral Pontine Syndrome....78
FIGURE 13.1.108 - Region Affected by Anterior Cord Syndrome....80
FIGURE 13.1.109 - Region Affected by Central Cord Syndrome....80
FIGURE 13.1.110 - Region Affected by Brown-Sequard Syndrome....80
FIGURE 13.1.111 - Subdural Hematoma....83
FIGURE 13.1.112 - Bridging Veins....83
FIGURE 13.1.113 - CT Scan of the Head: Acute Subdural Hematoma....84
FIGURE13.1.114 - CT Scan of the Head: Chronic Subdural Hematoma....84
FIGURE 13.1.115 - Epidural Hematoma....84
FIGURE 13.1.116 - Pterion and Middle Meningeal Artery....84
FIGURE 13.1.117 - CT Scan of the Head: Epidural Hematoma....85
FIGURE 13.1.118 - Subarachnoid Hemorrhage....87
FIGURE 13.1.119 - CT Angiography: Berry Aneurysm....87
FIGURE 13.1.120 - MRI of the Brain: AV Malformation....87
FIGURE 13.1.121 - Circle of Willis....88
FIGURE 13.1.122 - CT Scan of the Head: Subarachnoid Hemorrhage....88
FIGURE 13.1.123 - CTA: Subarachnoid Hemorrhage and Arterial Aneurysm....88
FIGURE 13.1.124 - Xanthochromia....88
FIGURE 13.1.125 - Intraparenchymal Hemorrhage....89
FIGURE 13.1.126 - CT Scan of the Head: Intracerebral Hemorrhage....89
FIGURE 13.1.127 - Intracranial Hemorrhage....90
FIGURE 13.1.128 - Visual Aura....91
FIGURE 13.1.129 - Mechanism of Action of Triptans....91
FIGURE 13.1.130 - Types of Primary Headache....92
FIGURE 13.1.131 - Light Microscopy of Rosenthal Fibers in Pilocytic Astrocytoma....95
FIGURE 13.1.132 - MRI of the Brain: Pilocytic Astrocytoma....95
FIGURE 13.1.133 - Pilocytic Astrocytoma....96
FIGURE 13.1.134 - Light Microscopy showing Pseudopalisading Necrosis in Glioblastoma Multiforme....96
FIGURE 13.1.135 - MRI of the Brain: Glioblastoma Multiforme....96
FIGURE 13.1.136 - Glioblastoma Multiforme....96
FIGURE 13.1.137 - Light Microscopy Showing Fried-Egg Appearance in Oligodendroglioma....99
FIGURE 13.1.138 - MRI Displaying Oligodendroglioma....99
FIGURE 13.1.139 - Light Microscopy: Perivascular Pseudorosettes in Ependymoma....99
FIGURE 13.1.140 - MRI of the Brain: Ependymoma....99
FIGURE 13.1.141 - Light Microscopy: Antoni A Pattern in Schwannoma....101
FIGURE 13.1.142 - Light Microscopy: Antoni B Pattern in Schwannoma....101
FIGURE 13.1.143 - MRI of the Brain: Schwannoma....101
FIGURE 13.1.144 - Light Microscopy: Homer Wright Rosettes in Medulloblastoma....102
FIGURE 13.1.145 - MRI of the Brain: Medulloblastoma....102
FIGURE 13.1.146 - Light Microscopy: Hemangioblastoma....102
FIGURE 13.1.147 - MRI of the Brain: Hemangioblastoma....103
FIGURE 13.1.148 - Light Microscopy: Psammoma Body in Meningioma....104
FIGURE 13.1.149 - MRI of the Brain: Meningioma....104
FIGURE 13.1.150 - The Pituitary Gland....104
FIGURE 13.1.151 - The Sella Turcica....104
FIGURE 13.1.152 - The Optic Pathway....105
FIGURE 13.1.153 - Light Microscopy: Cells of Pituitary Adenoma....105
FIGURE 13.1.154 - Light Microscopy: Craniopharyngioma....105
FIGURE 13.1.155 - MRI of the Brain: Pituitary Adenoma....105
FIGURE 13.1.156 - MRI of the Brain: Craniopharyngioma....106
FIGURE 13.1.157 - CT Scan of the Head: Metastatic Brain Tumors....106
FIGURE 13.1.158 - Inner Ear....109
FIGURE 13.1.159 - MRI of the Brain: Acoustic Neuroma....109
FIGURE 13.1.160 - Bell's Palsy....109
FIGURE 13.1.161 - Dix-Hallpike Maneuver....110
FIGURE 13.1.162 - Head Thrust Test....110
FIGURE 13.1.163 - Decreased Skin Turgor....113

Made in United States
Troutdale, OR
10/01/2026

55033281R00071